How to feed your family

Your one-stop guide to creating
healthy meals everyone will enjoy

CHARLOTTE STIRLING-REED

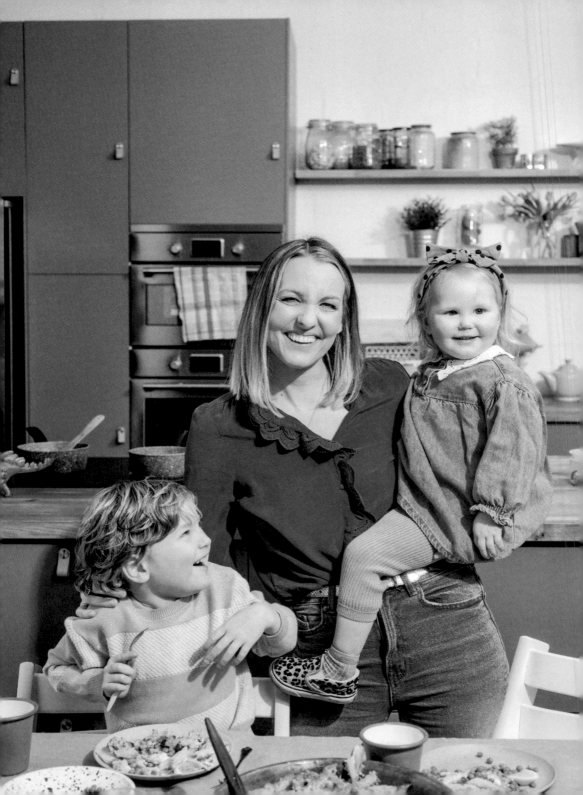

CONTENTS

INTRODUCTION   4

1 Your Family's Nutrition   10

2 Family Mealtimes   40

3 Getting Organised   56

4 Recipes   102

INDEX   222
ACKNOWLEDGEMENTS   224

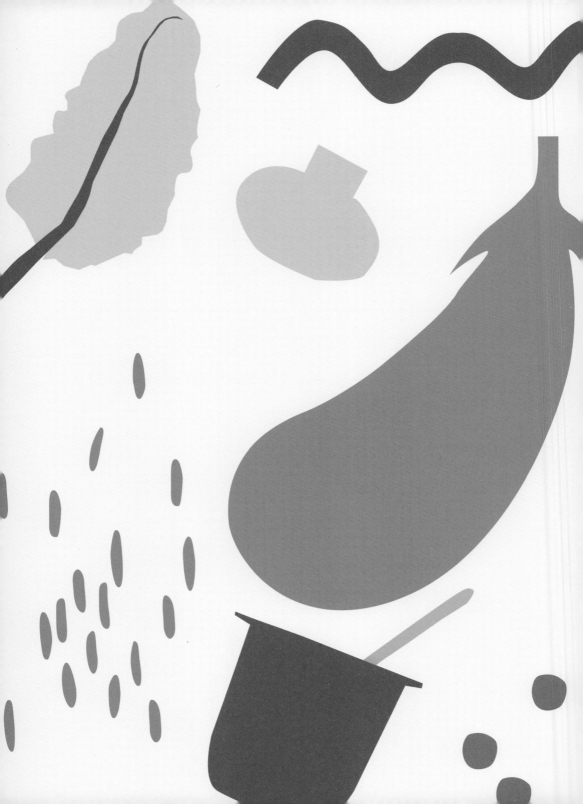

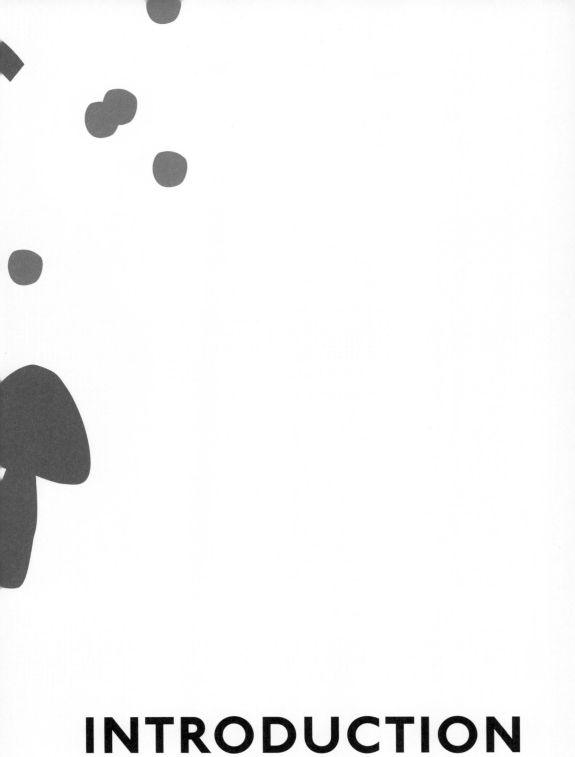

INTRODUCTION

Welcome to my new book – it has been such a joy to write!

While *How to Wean Your Baby* was all about taking your baby from their very first foods right through to eating family meals, and *How to Feed Your Toddler* covered everything to help you navigate that tricky period when toddlerhood kicks in and everything you thought you knew about parenting is no longer working, this book is a little bit different.

How to Feed Your Family aims to support you with everything you need to know about feeding, cooking and prepping meals for the whole family, however many children you have!

When I started writing this book, I was really in the thick of it all – school holidays, the 'terrible twos', juggling a career, family and home, and everything in between. With this book, I wanted to create a toolkit for parents – a bible almost – to make feeding families easier, taking some pressure off, offering meal ideas, inspiration and hacks that can really help at home, but at the same time acknowledging that it doesn't always have to be perfect … sometimes your best will do.

How to Feed Your Family is less about the psychology of eating or the 'do's and don'ts' of feeding kids, and much more about the excitement, organisation and skills you can utilise when cooking and prepping food at home. Of course, it also has a nutrition element to it, as I know how much families care about feeding their children (and themselves) a healthy, balanced diet. This book contains a whole chapter about what and how to feed your family, to offer the nutrition that we all need to be healthy and get in the right vitamins and minerals every day.

Helping your whole family to eat well and follow a healthy diet can seem like an unachievable aim, especially when everyone is so very busy – different schedules, classes, school times, working hours, bedtimes – and let's not forget sleepless nights! Throw on top of that needing to make different meals for everyone and food refusal, and you can see why mealtimes can become a drain, and why we reach for quick-and-easy takeaways and frozen meals (which is absolutely fine to do, by the way!).

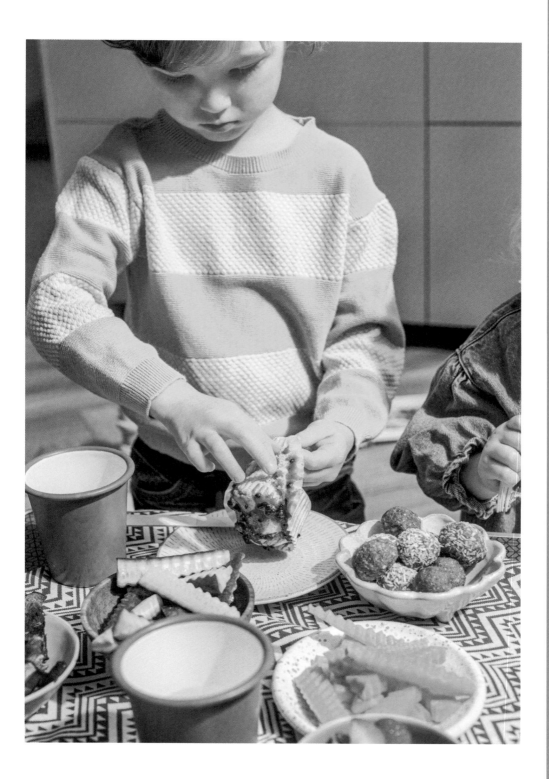

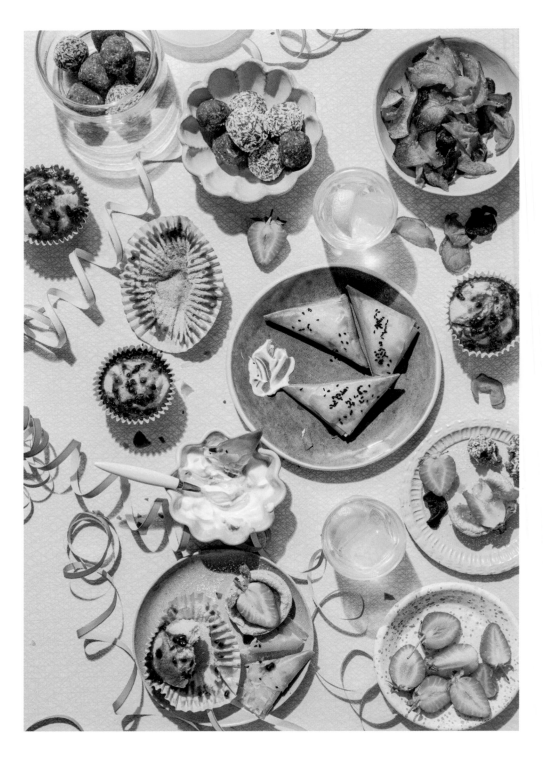

We often have a multitude of obstacles in our way, preventing us from creating delicious meals that are happily gobbled up:

Time: many of us struggle to fit it all in, cooking, cleaning and prepping food.

Stress: often the last thing you feel like doing is cooking meals from scratch for the whole family. Stress can really take the enjoyment out of so many things.

Work life: when you're exhausted from a day at work, it can be tough to build the motivation and energy needed to cook.

Budget: there's a misconception that eating well has to be expensive.

Access: getting access to the foods you want can be tricky, especially if you don't drive or you need specialist ingredients.

Complexity in dietary needs: sometimes you might feel limited in what food options you can choose due to allergies or dietary restrictions.

Different preferences: it can be hard to choose meals that everyone will enjoy.

Family eating at different times: different schedules and routines may make it hard for you to eat together and you might find yourself making multiple meals.

Food refusal and meal-skipping: this can make mealtimes a battleground and it can feel futile to create meals for fussy eaters!

If you regularly come across some of these obstacles, please know that it's OK and you're not alone. As a parent myself, I constantly feel like I'm 'failing' or not doing enough, and sometimes this can make you feel disheartened and demotivated. Part of the reason I wanted to write this book was to help myself and my own family, to hone my tips and make healthy eating as a family more practical and enjoyable. I hope that this book will get you excited about offering delicious, healthy, energy-giving food to your family much more easily and practically. Writing this book has really helped me to enjoy cooking more, feed my own family healthier food, while also reducing food waste and having fun with ingredients. I hope it does the same for you. I can't wait for you to read it and to see you utilising the tips and trying out the recipes too!

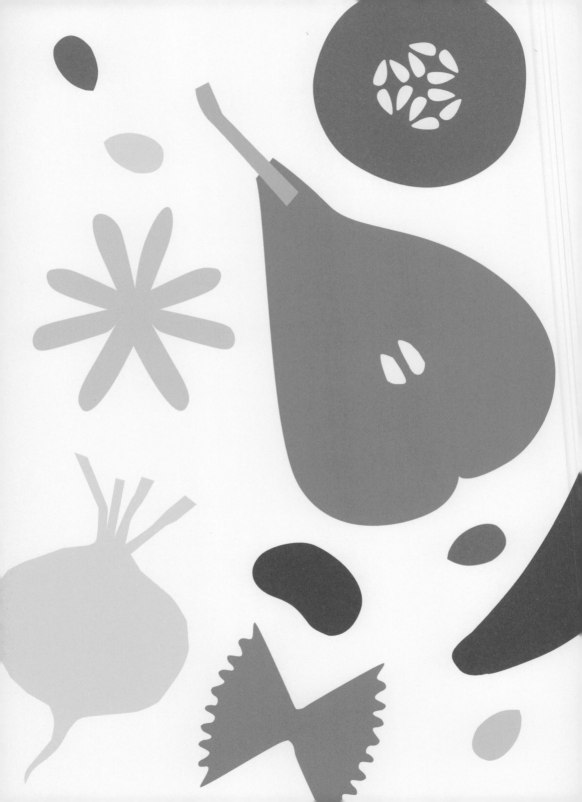

1

YOUR FAMILY'S NUTRITION

When it comes to working out how to feed your family a healthy, balanced diet, you first need to know the basics. This chapter covers everything you need to know about achieving that all-important 'balance' in family meals and getting the nutrition right.

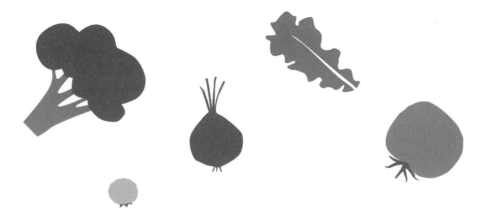

Nutrition really matters; what we eat helps support our bodies, reduces ill health, gives us energy and makes us feel better mentally as well as physically. For growing children it's so important too, to help them lay down the best foundations possible. Children are little sponges, and what happens in the home, seeing their parents and caregivers having a healthy relationship with food, is likely to have a positive impact on their own diets in the long run. So how we feed our families and how we talk about and enjoy foods together really makes a difference.

It can be so hard to 'get it all right', but the truth is that no one is perfect, and no one gets it right all of the time. So, if your toddler hasn't eaten a decent meal in days, or your teenager isn't eating at home with you, or your partner is not in line with your parenting messages, or nursery is offering jelly and ice cream regularly – it's OK. It's what happens the majority of the time that matters.

Healthy Eating Recommendations

When it comes to 'healthy eating' recommendations, guidelines vary globally, but most focus on offering an eating pattern that is similar to the recommendations below.

A balanced diet helps us to consume enough calories, proteins, fats, carbohydrates and vitamins and minerals to function and live a healthy life day to day. It's maybe too challenging to individually count the nutrients in your meals each day to ensure that you get, say, 14.8mg of iron or that you're having at least 45g of protein. Therefore, the recommendations outlined here show a representation of what a diet that offers all those nutrients in the right proportions might look like.

It doesn't have to be perfect every day, and I guarantee it won't be, but if you can feed your family meals that contain a variety and look roughly like the balance shown here most of the time, you're doing a great job!

These guidelines also encourage variety as a key element of a balanced diet. Different foods (even within the same food groups) contain a variety of nutrients that help to make up a balanced diet. For example, if you only ate bananas from the fruit and veg food group, you wouldn't be getting the 'balance' of nutrients you need.

The following guide explains the recommendation for most people over the age of two. However, under two years of age the recommendation is to loosely follow a similar pattern from weaning age, in smaller proportions (with a few small differences), but largely moving towards a 'balanced diet' as shown here so that babies and young children are getting a balance of what they need.

Around a third of food consumed per day should be carbohydrates, with a focus on wholegrains – including wholegrain breads, oats, pasta, rice, couscous, quinoa, potatoes, rye, chapatti, cereals, barley, noodles, freekeh and cassava. Vary the types offered. Some members of the family will need more carbohydrates and others less, depending on growth and energy levels.

Important for providing energy, protein and also fibre. These foods are also a good source of B vitamins and often include minerals such as calcium, zinc, folate and magnesium.

For specific recommendations for this food group referring to babies, see page 29.

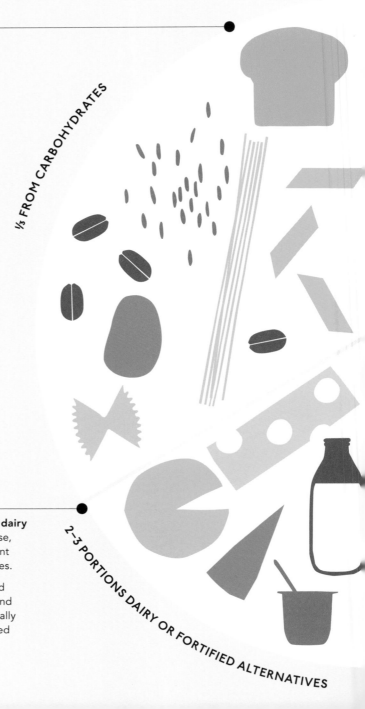

⅓ FROM CARBOHYDRATES

2–3 PORTIONS DAIRY OR FORTIFIED ALTERNATIVES

2–3 portions of dairy or fortified dairy alternatives a day, including cheese, yoghurt, milk, custard, fortified plant drinks, fortified yoghurt and cheeses.

Important for providing protein and calcium, as well as other vitamins and minerals such as B vitamins (especially B12) and iodine. Choose unflavoured varieties.

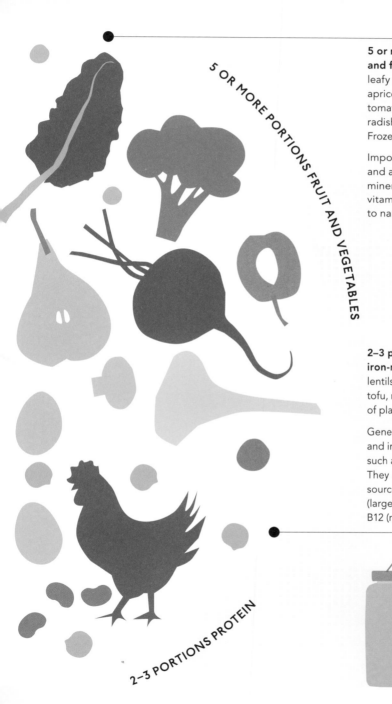

5 OR MORE PORTIONS FRUIT AND VEGETABLES

2–3 PORTIONS PROTEIN

5 or more portions of vegetables and fruits a day, e.g., green leafy veggies, carrots, peas, okra, apricots, peppers, apples, pears, tomatoes, berries, cabbage, radishes. Vary the types offered. Frozen and tinned qualify, too.

Important for providing fibre and a variety of vitamins and minerals, including vitamin C, vitamin A, folate and potassium, to name a few!

2–3 portions of protein- and iron-rich foods a day, e.g., beans, lentils, chickpeas, meat, fish, eggs, tofu, nuts and seeds. Offer plenty of plant-based proteins.

Generally, these contain protein and iron as well as minerals such as zinc and magnesium. They are also generally a good source of omega-3 fatty acids (largely from fish) and vitamin B12 (meat sources).

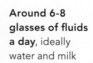

Around 6-8 glasses of fluids a day, ideally water and milk

Ways to easily balance family meals

When you're creating meals for your family, use the handy guide below to help you balance most meals and therefore include the majority of nutrients, vitamins and minerals you need each day.

Here are some examples of how to balance your family's meals:

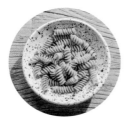 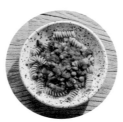 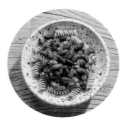 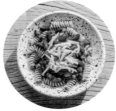

Start with a carb, e.g., some wholegrain pasta.

Add some fruit or veg, e.g., a veggie pasta sauce with tomatoes, courgette and peas.

Add some protein-/ iron-rich foods, e.g., kidney beans or some beef mince.

Sometimes add some dairy or dairy-free alternatives, e.g., grated cheese.

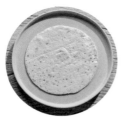 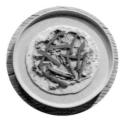 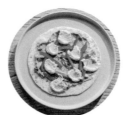 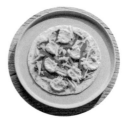

Start with a carb, e.g., a wrap.

Add some fruit or veg, e.g., avocado, pepper sticks and some orange segments (on the side).

Add some protein-/ iron-rich foods, e.g., hummus or strips of chicken.

Sometimes add some dairy or dairy-free alternatives, e.g., a dollop of yoghurt or some grated cheese.

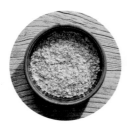 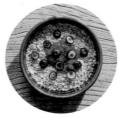 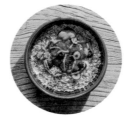 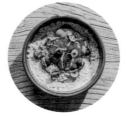

Start with a carb, e.g., oats.

Add some fruit or veg, e.g., mixed berries or chopped fruit.

Add some protein-/ iron-rich foods e.g., nut butter/ milled seeds.

Sometimes add some dairy or dairy-free alternatives, e.g., fortified plant milk or plant-based yoghurt.

Other Important Things to Consider for Balanced Family Nutrition

FIVE (AT LEAST) A DAY

Many of us don't eat enough fruit and veg, so it's a good idea to try to include a variety. Even small 'palm-sized' portions count towards this and it can be so simple to add them at each snack and meal occasion.

Beans and pulses count towards fruit and veg intakes, but only once. They do contain fibre and vitamins and minerals, but the levels and types of these are not the same as those found in other fruits and vegetables.

Juices count, but also just once as some of the fibre is lost in the blending process. Sugars are much more readily available and broken down into simple sugars in juices. It's best to dilute juices for one- to five-year-olds if offering.

VARIETY

The more variety you offer, the more kids become 'familiar' with different options, ensuring they get all those important nutrients. If you're ever worried about whether they've had 'too much' of anything, just come back to thinking about variety. Variety can take the pressure off: if you're worried they're having too much milk, swap a cup of milk for a different snack, such as veg sticks and hummus; or having eggs every day, swap some for a bean salad or other plant-based proteins such as chickpeas, tofu, lentils or nut butters.

FLUIDS

It's easy to get into a habit of offering sweet or calorie-rich drinks to the family, but one of the best and biggest changes you can make to your family's diet is offering more water for hydration and replacing sweet and sugary drink options with water. You can go cold turkey, slowly reduce sugary drink options in the family home or opt for alternatives such as diluted juice or infused water. Remember, milk and water are the only tooth-friendly options for young children.

FATS

Fats are important to include, so don't be afraid to cook with oil and use unsalted spreads, but try to choose healthier cooking oils where possible (see pages 94–95). Including healthy fats in your family's diet, such as olive oil, oily fish, avocado, nuts and seeds, is also a great way to offer extra energy and some essential fats along with a variety of nutrients too, which is especially important for growing babies and young children.

What Are Nutrients?

When it comes to nutrients, it can be helpful to know a bit more about why variety is so key.

Nutrients in our foods are broken down into macronutrients and mircronutrients:

Macronutrients

These are nutrients needed in larger quantities that provide our bodies with the energy it needs every day. They include fat, carbohydrates and proteins:

FAT	Provides plenty of calories and is important for the lining of body cells as well as helping to supply stores of energy and nutrients. Fat helps in the absorption of fat-soluble vitamins too.
CARBOHYDRATES	Provide a readily available source of energy for the body and contain fibre which is important for digestion.
PROTEINS	Important building blocks for growth and development and the immune system.

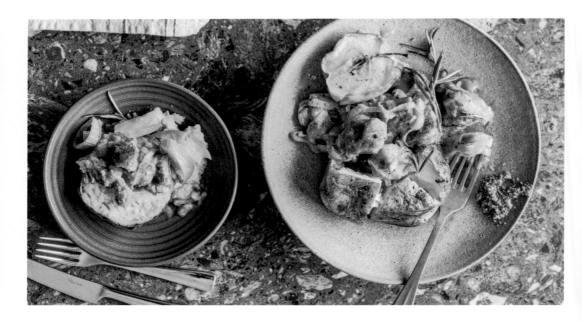

Micronutrients

These are nutrients we need in smaller quantities but are equally important in our diets and are largely made up of vitamins and minerals. These are not all the nutrients in our foods – there are plenty more, including important plant compounds such as phytonutrients and antioxidants – but these are some of key ones:

VITAMIN A	Important for the immune system and for healthy vision. Also helps in the protective function of the skin.
VITAMIN C	Important for the immune and nervous systems, and also protecting the body's cells from damage as vitamin C is also an antioxidant. Vitamin C helps to form collagen which is needed for bones, teeth and skin.
VITAMIN D	Not something that we can get huge amounts of from food, but vitamin D is important for supporting the body to absorb calcium from food and helps with muscle function and our immune system.
VITAMIN E	An antioxidant which helps to protect the body's cells against damage.
VITAMIN K	Needed to support blood clotting in the body and also for the structure of bones.
B VITAMINS	A group of vitamins which have a variety of essential roles throughout the body, including helping to break down the energy from food and helping with nervous system function and the creation of red blood cells.
CALCIUM	Best known for keeping our bones and teeth healthy, especially important for growing children and pregnant women, as well as reducing the impact of ageing on our bones. Also needed for the normal functioning of nerves and muscles.
FOLATE	Important for creating red blood cells and also reducing tiredness as well as supporting the immune and nervous systems.
IODINE	Important for brain function and development, supports hormone production from the thyroid which is essential for many other processes within the body.
IRON	Important for brain and immune function, but also for the creation of healthy red blood cells to help provide oxygen to cells around the body.
MAGNESIUM	Helps with nerve function and maintaining strong bone health. Also plays a role in releasing energy from our foods.
PHOSPHORUS	Similar to magnesium, important for nerve function and the release of energy from foods.
ZINC	Supports maintenance of skin, hair and nails, and helps with wound healing as well as brain function. Also contributes to normal fertility and reproduction.
SELENIUM	Helps to protect the cells in our bodies against damage. It also supports the immune system and helps maintain normal skin and nails, and normal fertility in males.
POTASSIUM	Helps regulate water content in the body and maintain normal blood pressure. It also helps nerves and muscles function effectively.

Sugar, salt and saturated fat

These are nutrients that we're recommended to eat less of, largely because having too much of them can have negative effects on our health in the long term.

Sugar is easy to eat in excess, so if we're having lots of sweet foods, we could end up consuming more calories than we need, which may lead to excess weight, high blood pressure and the risk of health conditions such as diabetes.

Salt has been linked to high blood pressure and cardiovascular disease, so it's important not to have high intakes over time, especially for people who are more susceptible to high blood pressure and cardiovascular disease. Salt shouldn't be added to young children's food.

It's best to try and **swap saturated fats** in the diet (which come in foods such as cakes, biscuits and pastries) for healthier fats such as mono and polyunsaturated fats that have benefits in the human body and come with plenty of vitamins and minerals too. Healthier fats are found in foods such as avocado, oily fish, nuts and seeds and olive oil.

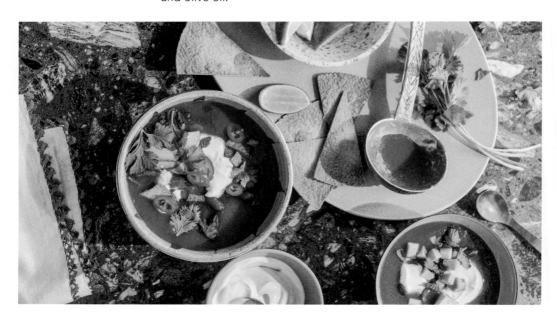

Processed foods

It's absolutely fine to eat processed foods, and many of the foods we eat day to day, such as tinned tomatoes, bread and pasta, are in some way processed. Ideally, no foods should be 'banned' in your family's diet (except for medical/cultural reasons). However, foods that are more highly processed (sometimes called ultra-processed foods) – such as crisps, biscuits, ham and sausages – tend to contain more in the way of sugar, salt and saturated fats and quite often have fewer of the nutrients we want to eat more of, so it's worthwhile trying to reduce your family's intake of heavily processed foods.

It's actually easier to do this than you might think:

 Cook many meals from scratch and avoid adding salt/sugars where possible.

 Check the back of packets and choose options with lower sugars/ salts and saturated fats where possible.

 Use a variety of ingredients in cooking, for example opt for different oils, low-salt spreads and butters, rather than just using salted butter whenever you cook.

 Choose quality meats and use less of them. Bulk out meals with plant-based proteins instead.

 Use herbs and spices when cooking to flavour foods, or use ingredients such as lemon juice to add flavour, instead of relying on salt and sugars alone.

 Use the label reading guide on page 87 to help you navigate food labels and choose healthier options for your family.

What Your Family Needs

In this section we're going to take a look at what different members of the family might need in their diet where it differs from the very general recommendations outlined above. Please note that this is very general advice, and if you're ever worried, it's worthwhile trying to chat to a healthcare professional directly to get some specific, tailored guidance.

Adults

Looking after our health as adults is often lower on our agenda, and it shouldn't be! As parents or carers, we have to make sure that we give ourselves enough energy and nutrients to help us deal with the day-to-day challenges of running a family, parenting and looking after everyone else's needs! You can't pour from an empty cup, as they say.

The human body is incredible, but we only have one and we really need to look after it, keep it functioning to the best of its ability and for as long as possible. This means giving it enough calories, the right balance of macro- and micronutrients, and enough water to keep us hydrated, as well as plenty of rest and play!

Recommendations on the levels of nutrients or calories we need (2,000kcal for women and 2,500kcal for men, for example) are just guidelines – we're all individual and so our needs are often very different. If you're in a larger body and you're more active, you may need more in the way of portions, calories and nutrients than someone who is smaller and who is less active, for example.

However, there are some areas where we are generally falling short and where we might need to focus to ensure we're getting enough of everything.

Generally, adults are:

✗	not eating enough oily fish
✗	eating too much red and processed meat (especially men)
✗	not eating enough fruits and vegetables
✗	not consuming enough fibre
✗	eating too many free sugars

We can try to change this by:

✓	Opting for oily fish once a week, or including foods such as walnuts, flaxseeds, enriched eggs, olive oil or an algae omega-3 supplement in our diet.
✓	Including meat but eating less of it and choosing better quality. Bulking out meals with lentils, beans or pulses instead.
✓	Adding fruits and veggies to every meal and having them as snacks through the day. For example, add dried fruits or frozen berries to breakfast, take mini cucumbers or carrot sticks with a dip to snack on at work, have a side salad with lunch and add beans and pulses to whatever you're cooking in the evening.
✓	Choosing wholegrains where possible, swapping white bread/pasta/rice for brown options. If that's too hard, try going for half and half when making meals and snacks.
✓	Trying to eat less sugar (no need to cut it out entirely!) and snack on fruits instead. Frozen grapes and berries, dried apricots and fresh figs make for good sweet replacements. Choose lower-sugar sweets and cereals and add your own sweetness with fruits at home where you can.

Additional needs for adults

Women especially (but not solely) are also falling short on a few important vitamins and minerals. These include:

OMEGA-3 FATTY ACIDS

Most men and women aren't eating enough oily fish to help them get important healthy fats such as omega-3. It's good to try to include one portion of oily fish in your diet a week if you eat fish. If not, other sources such as fortified foods (spreads, eggs and breakfast cereals), walnuts, olive oil, flaxseeds and tofu can be alternatives. If you don't eat many or enough of these foods, then think about taking an omega-3/ algae supplement.

Women of childbearing age (who want to have children or more children at some point) are recommended to have no more than two portions of oily fish a week and men/general population are recommended to have no more than four, due to small levels of pollutants that oily fish can contain.

IRON

Women have higher requirements due to menstruation, especially if they aren't getting enough iron-rich foods or have very heavy periods. Many people don't know that iron supplements are actually recommended for women who have heavy periods regularly (check with your GP or pharmacist for more details).

FIBRE

Both men and women fall short when it comes to including enough fibre in their diet. Eating regular meals, including wholegrains, and getting five or more fruits and veggies in your diet should help here. With fibre, it's often really simple to make some changes to up the amount you're having.

Wholegrains are foods that retain the whole part of the grain and haven't had any of their nutritious elements stripped. These include oats, wholegrain bread, pasta and brown rice. Eating more wholegrains will help to increase fibre intake.

CALCIUM

Another important nutrient as women are at higher risk of osteoporosis and can have calcium losses during pregnancy, especially if they haven't consumed enough or didn't have enough pre-pregnancy stores. Not everyone needs a supplement, but eating enough calcium-rich foods can help.

FOLATE

For women of childbearing age, folic acid supplements are recommended to be taken from when they decide they want to have a baby until the twelfth week of pregnancy.

Supplements

There aren't really any specific supplements you need to take as adults, with the exception of vitamin D.

Vitamin D is needed for some really important functions in the body, including helping with the absorption of calcium, the maintenance of bones and muscles, and the normal functioning of the immune system. A supplement of 10mcg of vitamin D is recommended to be taken by all adults from October to April, when we simply don't make enough vitamin D from the sun, and you could consider taking one all year round. It's recommended to take a supplement containing 10mcg of vitamin D all year for those who:

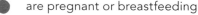 are pregnant or breastfeeding
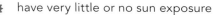 have very little or no sun exposure
are not often outdoors – for example, are frail, housebound or in a care home
usually wear clothes that cover up most of their skin when outdoors
have dark skin – for example, have an African, African-Caribbean or south Asian background

Consider other specific supplements or a general multivitamin if you:

 Have a limited diet or don't eat a balanced diet (see pages 14–15).

 Are a little fussy and picky with your own food.

 Are vegetarian. Consider supplements that include iron, vitamin B12 and omega-3 or opt for fortified foods.

Are vegan. Consider supplements that include iodine, iron, omega-3, vitamin B12, zinc, selenium and calcium or opt for fortified foods which contain these.

 Don't eat fish. Consider an algae omega-3 supplement or eat plenty of omega-3 fortified foods.

 Are on any other restrictive diet. It might be helpful to have a chat with a pharmacist or healthcare professional about what (if any) supplements might be useful for you to take.

It isn't always easy being a parent or carer and it can be exhausting. Below are some tips to help you look after yourself amidst the chaos at home:

TAKE TIME FOR YOUR MEALS. Eating mindfully gives you some breathing space in the day and helps your digestive system work more efficiently. How many of us are eating meals on the go, while doing the washing or getting in the car with the kids? Try to build mindful meals into your week and properly enjoy your food.

STAY HYDRATED. It's so easy to pack a bottle for the kids and forget one for you! Aim for 6–8 glasses of water a day, or at least drink enough to keep your urine diluted.

TIPS FOR BUSY

GIVE YOURSELF ENOUGH ENERGY. Skipping meals, forgetting to eat, picking bits off the kids' plates and calling it lunch … Sound familiar? This isn't ideal for parents/carers who need to be on top of their energy levels. Our energy comes from our food and, if we're not properly fuelling ourselves throughout the day, it's going to add to those feelings of tiredness, exhaustion, lack of motivation or feeling a little low. We must prioritise fuelling ourselves in order for us to fuel our kids too.

Iron, folate, magnesium and B vitamins will help to reduce fatigue, while protein, iron, B vitamins, folate and vitamin C are important for supporting the immune system (which may be low in fatigued and sleep-deprived parents/carers).

STICK TO A ROUTINE. This allows you to get enough of everything you need. Listen to your own hunger and fullness cues rather than only focusing on feeding your kids (guilty!). People have different patterns of eating, but something similar to three main meals and two snacks might be helpful.

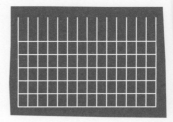

GET ORGANISED WITH MEALS. Order food shopping online and stock your freezer with batch-cooked dishes. It'll make such a difference. If you can, write out meal plans for the week and use these to help you reduce food waste and to take the brainwork out of meals (see pages 74–77). Don't forget to ask for help from those who offer – asking someone to cook you some meals, or babysit while you batch cook, can make a big difference to the rest of your week.

GET SOME REST. Easier said than done, but one of the ways we can recuperate, recharge and repair properly is giving ourselves rest time. Tap into offers of help, take a 30-minute nap instead of cleaning the bathroom, or make the most of nights off. Allowing yourself time to rest can be so key to giving you the motivation and headspace to deal with everything as a parent/carer.

PARENTS/ CARERS

MOVE, DON'T FOCUS ON 'EXERCISE'. What do you enjoy? Pottering in the garden? Walking with your baby in the pram or sling? A stroll around a park with a friend? Getting active with your toddler? A 10-minute power walk to the shops? Life with kids is pretty fast-paced anyway, so you'll probably find that you're a lot more active than you think!

I remember when I was postpartum with my daughter and kept reading everywhere about getting back into exercise and it was the furthest from anything I wanted to do. It took me a long while to do anything substantial, as physically and emotionally I'd taken a bit of a hit, but then I realised that exercise can be what I make of it – even chatting on the phone while walking around the house with Ada strapped to me, or dancing around the kitchen, for example.

HAVE YOU:	Monday	Tuesday	Wednesday	Thursday	Friday	Saturday	Sunday
HAD 5+ FRUIT AND VEG?							
HAD 3–5 SERVINGS OF WHOLE GRAINS?							
HAD 2–3 SERVINGS OF PROTEINS/IRON?							
HAD 2–3 DAIRY OR DAIRY-FREE ALTERNATIVES?							
HAD 6–8 GLASSES OF FLUID?							
DONE SOME MOVEMENT/ EXERCISE?							
TAKEN YOUR VITAMIN D/ SUPPLEMENT?							

Use this chart to help remind you of the basics you need to look after yourself and your health. Don't worry if you miss some on some days; just use this checklist as a gentle reminder of what you need to look after you! Visit **www.srnutrition.co.uk** for a downloadable copy of this.

Babies and toddlers

Babies and toddlers do have different requirements. They need:

 A higher fat diet as they are growing at a fast rate and need plenty of calories.

 Lots of energy and energy-dense foods.

 Lots of nutrients relative to their small body size, so the foods they eat need to be packed with nutrition.

 Smaller portions than adults.

To avoid or limit certain foods, or have their food prepped in certain ways.

Food textures adapted for them until they are older and have developed their oral motor skills efficiently.

Greater amount of milk as an energy and nutrient source, up to 12 months of age.

0–12 MONTHS

Under six months, breast or formula milk is all babies need to grow and develop. Once weaning starts, food gradually starts to become a more important source of calories and nutrients, but also in helping little ones learn about eating. This doesn't mean milk has to stop – breastfeeding can be continued responsively for as long as you and your baby/toddler wish. After 12 months, if formula feeding, you can move on to full-fat cow's milk instead.

From around six months, babies will start learning about food and working on the skills and abilities needed to eat solid foods.

Between nine and twelve months, babies will move on to more 'adult-style' diets, eating more complex meals and having routines around their mealtimes. Ideally, they'll eat a wide variety of textures and foods. But there are still some foods that babies and toddlers need to avoid (see also page 83).

Foods that toddlers need to limit or avoid:

 Fibre: when it comes to white versus wholegrain carbohydrates, it's best to offer half and half to babies and toddlers up to two.

Sugar and salt are best avoided. Little ones just don't need them and, ideally, we don't want to encourage a taste and preference for these foods early on.

 Salty foods such as olives and smoked salmon should be offered in very small amounts. Foods such as processed and salty meats (like ham and pastrami) should be avoided for young toddlers until they are a little older and can have them in moderation.

1–4 YEARS

Other than the foods listed above, most other family foods are fine to offer in your little one's diet, and it's great to get them used to all the tastes and flavours of your home cooking. These meals might need slight adaptations, such as a little extra chopping or cooking a little softer, or not adding too much in the way of spicy heat.

During toddlerhood, fussy eating and food refusal can rear their heads. This is perfectly normal, but it can be a real challenge when it comes to mealtime peace.

Please try to remember that fluctuations in appetite are normal in children, and such a wide range of factors will impact their eating day to day. However, some things you can stick to as a family to help make food refusal just a phase include:

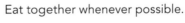 Role model eating a balanced diet.

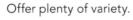 Eat together whenever possible.

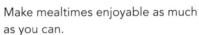 Offer plenty of variety.

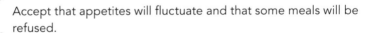 Make mealtimes enjoyable as much as you can.

 Accept that appetites will fluctuate and that some meals will be refused.

 Offer some autonomy around mealtimes and avoid mealtime pressures to eat.

 Keep in mind that you decide what you cook and what goes on their plate; they decide how much of that they actually want to eat.

If you're ever worried about your toddler's eating and food refusal is going on for a long time or their weight is affected, it's always best to have a chat with your GP or health visitor.

SUPPLEMENTS FOR BABIES AND TODDLERS

For babies 0–1 who are breastfed, 8.5–10mcg of vitamin D is recommended daily.

For babies 0–1 who are formula fed, they don't need to have this until they are having less than 500ml of formula milk a day (as the formula already contains the added vitamin D they need). Once they are having less than this, they need 8.5-10mcg vitamin D a day too.

On top of this recommendation, breastfed and formula-fed babies (as long as formula-fed babies are having less than 500ml of formula) are recommended to have a supplement of vitamin A and C each day from six months of age, as a safeguard in case they aren't getting enough. Children 1–4 are recommended to have 10mcg of vitamin D a day throughout the year.

Aside from this, there are no other recommendations to routinely supplement, but if your little one has dietary restrictions such as multiple allergies, is vegan or vegetarian, or they are becoming increasingly fussy with their food, a multivitamin may be helpful as a safeguard alongside as much of a balanced diet as you can offer. It's always best to chat to a healthcare professional if you're unsure.

Some important nutrients that babies and toddlers may be more at risk of being short of include:

- iron (due to high requirements for growth)
- calcium (due to growing bones)
- iodine (especially if they don't eat dairy or fish)
- omega-3 (for growing brains)
- fat (because they need plenty of high-fat foods and calories when they are growing)

HAVE YOU:	Monday	Tuesday	Wednesday	Thursday	Friday	Saturday	Sunday
OFFERED 3 (BALANCED) MEALS?							
OFFERED MILK AND/OR SNACKS?							
OFFERED 2–3 PORTIONS OF PROTEINS/IRON?							
OFFERED A VARIETY OF FRUIT AND VEG?							
OFFERED 6–8 SMALL GLASSES OF FLUIDS?							
GIVEN VITAMIN D OR A, C + D, OR A MULTIVITAMIN?							

Use this chart to help remind you of the things your little ones need most days.
Don't worry if you forget on the odd days; just use this checklist to give you a nudge to remember some of the basics. You can download your own version on my website, to fill in:
www.srnutrition.co.uk

Older kids and teens

Generally, children over two are recommended to slowly move towards a diet that is similar to that depicted on page 14 as a 'balanced diet' and, by five years of age, most children and adult recommendations are similar.

However, there are still likely to be trials and tribulations when it comes to mealtimes as you move through these ages, with developing independence, outside influences and changing hormones and personalities as our kids grow up.

Food refusal is likely to come and go during this time, and you might find your children change their eating pattern as they age and as you become less influential in what they eat outside of the home.

One important factor when raising kids is to try to help them have a healthy pattern of eating when they are young (and within your home) as this is likely to help them continue to be more familiar with this style of eating in the long run – even if they do go through phases of refusal, rebelling or copying outside influences!

Food can be an important element of children growing up and plays a role in people's identity. One thing I try to stress is that what happens at home and what's happening the majority of the time, as well as what behaviours they see you modelling, is likely to have an impact and make a difference, even if it doesn't feel like it at the time.

From our national surveys in the UK, we can see that young children and teens:

- have low intakes of fruit and vegetables

- aren't getting enough fibre

- are eating too much in the way of sugar and soft sweet drinks

- often are not getting enough iron in their diet

Ideally, to help them achieve a balanced diet daily, they need to:

 Focus on water as their main form of hydration

 Eat meals regularly and avoid skipping them

 Eat plenty of fruits and veggies – try to get portions in when you can when they are home

 Have healthy snacks readily available and as 'the norm' where possible.

 Avoid restricting whole food groups by encouraging a 'balance and moderation' approach to all foods – nothing cut out or overly restricted (unless for medical or cultural reasons)

Some other important elements which may have an impact on your older children and teen's nutritional intakes might include:

FOOD AND MOOD

Food has such an influence on mood. Without enough energy, it's hard for children to focus and you might find them getting 'hangry' between meals or if they haven't eaten enough.

How can I help?

 Try to encourage a regular routine where you can and include snacks in between main meals. Children are growing and developing at a fast rate and need to fuel that growth, especially if they are fairly active.

 Offer a variety and ensure plenty of fats and carbohydrates are offered at mealtimes. Try to keep snacks nutrient-rich by making them 'mini meals'.

 Try to help them understand their own feelings by stating your own hunger, and asking them if they are hungry when they are feeling/behaving in a hangry manner.

DEVELOPING INDEPENDENCE

As older kids and teens develop independence, this may mean that they want to have more of a say in the things they eat, the places they eat. Outside influences are likely to creep in when it comes to food choices, and this isn't always a bad thing.

How can I help?

 Try to maintain the 'norm' at home: a stable routine, a similar pattern of eating and familiar foods offered so that our children know what to expect.

 Offer plenty of independence in other aspects of their lives – what they wear, what they play with, etc.

FOOD LANGUAGE

The language we use with older children and teens around this time is crucial. We want to build positive relationships with food and help create confident and independent children.

How can I help?

 Be aware of how you talk about yourself, your body and the food that you're eating.

 Avoid labelling foods as 'bad' or overly restricting calories and food groups.

 Try not to talk negatively about what they are eating and avoid pressuring them to eat a certain way, as this is likely to backfire.

Kicking off the day with a filling, nutrient-dense breakfast can help to keep your teen's brain fuelled and give them enough energy for their concentration throughout the day. It's one of the reasons I like to 'make the most' of breakfast (as well as other meals). Try to make it balanced with some seeds, or nut butters, and a piece of fruit alongside cereal or toast and perhaps a little milk or yoghurt, for example.

There are other things that parents/carers of older children and teens might be faced with, such as meal skipping, outside influences and body image. Below are some useful tips to help your older children and teens to (eventually) eat well:

- Encourage independence in their food choices and allow them to have their own preferences. Emphasise these as a way to encourage them to have their own autonomy around what they eat. If we instil this when they are young, they might be more inclined to listen to their own body's needs rather than copying others as they get older.

- Allow them to eat out and make their own choices (at parties, with friends, etc.), but carry on offering healthy meals at home.

- Experiment with new foods, flavours and options regularly so that having something 'different' is the norm.

- Talk about human bodies, what they need and how they are all different. Try to encourage confidence with body image. Role-model healthy body image messages and avoid restricting foods yourself, alongside caring about your health and what you're eating.

- Talk about why healthy eating is important more from a 'feeling good' perspective and from the point of view of 'taking care' of yourself, than focusing on body shape and aesthetics.

- Encourage routine around food intakes as a way of listening to our bodies and understanding hunger and fullness cues.

- Talk to them about how they feel when they miss meals instead of trying to coax them into eating.

- Teach skills, such as cooking, prepping and shopping, but also things like how to create a balanced plate of food and how to be savvy with food labels (see pages 16 and 87).

- Make healthy habits easy where you can. Offer on-the-go breakfasts, mini meals and easier snacks to grab and go. Make healthy food available, ready chopped, have a good stash of food in the freezer and bulk-make meals where you can so there is plenty around.

- Keep mealtimes light and enjoyable as much as you can. The more they are pressure-free and engaging, the more your children and teens will want to be a part of them.

HAVE THEY:	Monday	Tuesday	Wednesday	Thursday	Friday	Saturday	Sunday
HAD 3 MAIN MEALS?							
INCLUDED SOME HEALTHY SNACKS?							
HAD 5+ FRUIT AND VEG?							
HAD 3–5 SERVINGS OF WHOLEGRAINS?							
HAD 2–3 PORTIONS PROTEINS/IRON?							
HAD 2–3 DAIRY OR DAIRY-FREE ALTERNATIVES?							
HAD 6–8 GLASSES OF FLUID?							
DONE SOME MOVEMENT/ EXERCISE?							
TAKEN VITAMIN D/MULTIVITAMIN SUPPLEMENT?							

Use this chart to help remind you of the things your kids need most days. Don't worry if you forget on the odd days; just use this checklist to give you a nudge to remember some of the basics. You can download your own version on my website, to fill in: **www.srnutrition.co.uk**

Portion size recommendations are really challenging. Everyone has different needs, and each individual will likely have different requirements for certain macro- and micronutrients. It's therefore hard to have a 'one-size-fits-all' approach to what we should be eating.

Ultimately, it's about having a balanced diet and trying to eat to appetite as much as you can, and having a routine around meals can help with that.

There are some good visual guides that offer a very rough estimate to what a portion might look like for you as an adult or child. These visuals can be helpful when we're thinking about portions for everyone in the family, as hand sizes will be smallest for your littlest family members and largest for the adults.

PORTION SIZES FOR

A HANDFUL (CUPPED)

2x cupped handfuls is a portion for dried carbohydrates, such as couscous, pasta, rice and breakfast cereals.

About 2x cupped handfuls for dried lentils, beans and chickpeas.

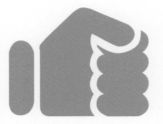

A FIST

A portion for a potato.

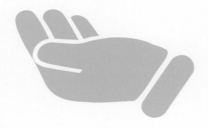

A PALM

A portion is 1x for most fish, steak and nuts and seeds.

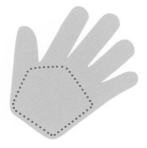

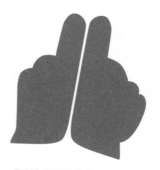

TWO THUMBS

A portion for cheese.

THE WHOLE FAMILY

THE WHOLE HAND SPREAD OUT

A portion is 1x for chicken and ½ for salmon and mackerel.

Remember these are estimates and it's really important to follow your young children's appetite cues as much as you can.

2

FAMILY MEALTIMES

I know all too well that the idea of a perfect family dinner with everyone smiling, together and happily eating their meals might seem a little far-fetched. In my house, mealtimes and prep are often chaotic, with kids clawing at my feet or having a tantrum while I'm cooking. Additionally, if 'family mealtimes' bring up reminders of arguing or battles to get kids to eat, you're certainly not alone. This is very common.

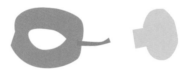

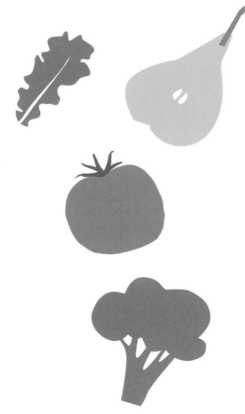

However, there is a lot of research on the benefits of family mealtimes, including an increase in the likelihood of children eating healthy foods. Research also suggests that family mealtimes can represent the idea of 'family togetherness', encourage communication and language skills in young children, offer opportunities for fun, learning about each other, and provide an opportunity to model and teach about healthy foods and having a positive relationship with food.

In this chapter, I want to show you that eating together and enjoying family mealtimes is possible, and doesn't have to end in disaster.

Mediterranean-style Eating

The Mediterranean style of eating is a key part of the advice I offer about family nutrition. This way of eating can offer huge benefits.

A lot of the advantages of a Mediterranean diet are around the specific dietary pattern and types of foods traditionally eaten in Mediterranean cultures. For example, there is a focus on plant foods and including foods such as nuts and seeds, fruits and veggies, plentiful olive oils as staples, as well as moderate amounts of fish, meat and dairy.

However, the Mediterranean diet offers much more than its nutritional benefits, and is more about:

- the way of eating

- eating meals together

- the environment in which food is eaten

- the process of creating meals from scratch

- taking time out for meals

- resting after meals

- conversation and nurturing one another at mealtimes

- interaction and the development of relationships around the table

- palatable, familiar and culturally appropriate foods on offer

- family communications

- everyone pausing for lunch

I love to talk about these two definitions that really help to sum up what the Mediterranean diet is really about (aside from the delicious food!):

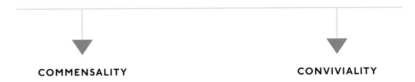

COMMENSALITY

the aspect of eating together with family and friends.

CONVIVIALITY

the social aspect of eating together, including socialising during meals and the pleasure of shared dishes together.

It's these definitions that set the Mediterranean diet apart. It's not about eating convenient, quick meals alone, but more about the way we think about, cook and eat our foods.

Having said all this, I know that it's not possible for many of us to come together every day to share meals as big families and communities; it's just not the way of the world anymore, and even in many Mediterranean countries now this often isn't common practice. But that doesn't mean we can't take aspects of the Mediterranean diet and try to bring them into our family food environment as and when we can.

I know that, with all the will in the world, this isn't going to be how many of us can serve our meals regularly, but anything you can do to just help that mealtime environment be more enjoyable – be more present, offer the kids more autonomy and help to build family relationships around meals – will be beneficial.

In my family, mealtimes are key to encouraging better eating and enjoyment of food. Don't get me wrong, we don't eat meals together every single day and certainly not at every mealtime, but, when we can, sitting together and eating similar foods can really help us to share a bit of joy around food as a family.

Here are some of the ways I try to do this in my day-to-day family life:

 Focus on a variety of delicious foods, largely plants.

 Eat together as a family whenever it's possible to do so.

 Have 'shared' meals as much as we can so the kids see us eating the same foods.

 Use mealtimes together as opportunities to bond, connect and learn about each other.

 Keep mealtimes as light and enjoyable occasions as much as possible.

 Offer platters of food and/or a 'buffet' of options and simply choose the bits that we want, and allow others to do the same.

 Try to make the environment pleasant, eating when everyone is calm and maybe playing some relaxing music to add to the ambience.

 Be kind and thoughtful around mealtimes and ask about each other's days.

 Invite friends around for meals more often and try to bring the kids to the table with us for occasions or when eating out too.

 Let little ones share in the pleasures of eating and show our enjoyment for mealtimes when we can.

 Get kids involved in the meals, serving, prepping, cooking and shopping to help them be part of the 'community' that brings meals together.

 Take the pressure off meals and instead make eating about the occasion, not what gets eaten.

Obstacles to Family Mealtimes

OBSTACLE	RECOMMENDATION
Lack of time	Try to take the pressure off and focus on one or two quality family meals throughout the week, and really enjoy them together. It doesn't have to be every day or every meal.
Busy + conflicting schedules	Try to nail down a day when most/all of you are at home, even if that ends up being breakfast once a week or dinner at the weekend.
Preparation time	If you can, prep meals ahead, make meals in bulk when you have a few spare hours and freeze, so you have whole meals ready to go (see pages 76–77). Or have 'buffet dinners' which require less prep.
Knowledge/skills	There are plenty of simple recipes out there if you're not confident in the kitchen. Meals don't have to be extravagant to be healthy and something as simple as beans on toast might be just what the family needs.
Shopping times	Try online food shopping and save your favourites so it's easy to click and order each time. Pick a slot in the week when you have time to put the food away.
Family feelings/ behaviours	Try to keep the meals fun and pressure-free – easier said than done, I know. Keep calm and try to make the main focus lightness and enjoyment – even if that means taking a step back and not focusing on food being eaten.
Lack of support	Ask for help. Get the kids involved in putting food away and cleaning up or even serving dishes if possible. It might be more work at first, but giving them little chores will not only help you but is great for their learning and skill development.
Clean up	Try to do it just once in the day and get others involved where possible.
Mealtime conflicts	Keep mealtimes light and have a 'positive vibes only' rule at the table.

Having Fun with Food as a Family

Food and nutrition is not all about eating … believe it or not. Helping your family enjoy food can be an important part of their learning and acceptance of foods, no matter your age!

Get your family involved in reading, writing, drawing, singing, cooking and playing with foods. My daughter loves to pretend she's going 'shopping' and takes a bag with her and comes back with various items from the kitchen; playing shops can really help kids to learn what food is, where we get it from and even what to do with it. My son also used to love playing with his Velcro fruit and veggies, which helped him to learn their names and familiarise him with certain foods. Throughout their childhood we made a real effort to include various books and songs that have food as a central theme.

My son also has a little corner of the garden where he's planted herbs, and he is often running off to get us various herbs when we're cooking in the summer. It's a lovely way to show where food comes from, familiarise children with ingredients and what they smell and taste like. A few ways to bring fun into foods with your little ones:

POTATO STAMPS WITH PAINT... you can use carrot tops to paint Jackson Pollock-style and even use fruits and veggies as stencils for drawing.

GET THEM COOKING – from little tasks like spreading and stirring to full-on baking recipes when they are older. The earlier you build those skills, the more able and familiar they'll be with food.

ENCOURAGE THEM TO TELL STORIES about fruits and veggies or write little books and include food and mealtimes in their stories.

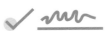

ASK THEM TO HELP YOU write (or draw) your shopping list and give them tasks to carry out at the supermarket.

GROW YOUR OWN: try indoor cress and other herbs, or outside have a tomato or strawberry plant for them to tend to.

MAKE A PRETEND SHOP at home and give them a little bag or trolley and let them play shops!

ASK THEM to wash all your fruits and veggies when you get them home from the shops.

PAINT AND DECORATE fruit/veg/egg shells and make pasta necklaces.

Encouraging Veggie Acceptance

Sometimes it's not just the youngest members of the family who struggle to eat veggies! And most of us could probably do with including more in our diet. On average, adults eat around 2–3 portions of fruits and veggies a day (the recommendation is really 5 as a minimum!) while older children between 11 and 18 years eat around 2.9 portions of fruit and veg a day.

Veggies are often tougher to get accepted by our kids than fruits, largely because children are born with a preference for sweeter foods and need some help and experience to learn to accept more bitter and savoury tastes that you get with a variety of vegetables.

We can certainly help our little ones to eat more and accept more veggies, but sometimes that starts with us – us offering it, us varying the types of veggies (and fruits) that they are given, and us eating them too … we are role models for our children so adopting a 'do as I do' approach is likely to help in the long run.

If you don't eat enough fruits and veggies yourself, try some of these tips for the whole family:

Have weekly 'new food' taste tests and get everyone in the family to rate the foods (you could even try doing this blind-folded!).

Spend some time in the fruit and veg aisle and look at all the varieties that are available, not just the ones you usually go for.

Offer small amounts of newish veggies alongside other well-accepted veggies – so if your little one loves peas, but hasn't had courgette often, offer plenty of peas and just one or two rounds of courgette to build familiarity.

Have a flick through a cookbook and try some new recipes with new veggie ingredients.

Add a dip alongside some simple veggie sticks – research shows that this helps kids accept and eat new veggies.

Think about ways to make your plates and meals more colourful – the more colours on the plate the better, nutritionally.

Serve veggies as a starter – this can be a good way of upping veggie intakes when everyone is hungry.

Don't forget about frozen veg – this is such a quick and easy way to add extra veg to meals and even as a snack.

Make them readily available, have batches of ready-to-eat veggie sticks in the fridge so they are easy to eat or take out and about with you.

Try family food charts where you get rewards for exploring, playing with or even just taking an interest in new foods and, once the chart is ticked off, you can do something nice together as a family.

Avoid pressuring anyone to eat veggies: simply offer them without comment.

Offer veggies in different ways – grated, raw, roasted, grilled, steamed or mashed, with herbs sprinkled on top.

Try mixing veggies (e.g. grated carrot, courgette and beetroot) into foods that you normally make – fritters, omelettes, cakes and bakes, porridge or muffins, and even add extra handfuls when cooking any of your main meals such as spag bol or curries – it can be a good way to up all of your intakes without much effort! Offer veggies at breakfast – in smoothies, granola or as a pancake topping (see recipes on pages 111 and 117).

Offer simple side salads along with main meals.

Food Language

The language we use at the table and around food can really impact how our children (and we) see mealtimes, eating and foods.

INSTEAD OF...	TRY... ♥
Talking about foods as 'good' or 'bad'	Name foods as they are: ice cream, not 'treat', and broccoli rather than 'healthy'
Offering certain foods as 'rewards' e.g. 'If you do that you can have dessert'	Avoid focusing on food rewards and offer other rewards, such as family time or playing a game together
Pressuring to eat	Take the attention away from the food and ask questions about their day
'It's delicious, try it'	Simply model eating and enjoying it yourself
'Please eat, I just made that for you'	Offer smaller portions and employ the phrase 'That's OK, you don't have to eat it'
'Please just have one more bite'	'That's OK, listen to your tummy and stop when you're full'
'I'm going on a diet'	'I need to eat more veggies'
'I ate way too much'	'I didn't listen to my tummy and now I'm over full!'
'What's wrong with it? You ate it yesterday'	'OK. What was the best thing you did at school today?'
'OK, well what do you want instead then?'	'I'm sorry, that's all that's on the menu tonight, but maybe we can have that next week?'

Food Refusal at the Table

Food refusal is very normal and often a standard part of raising children, so try not to worry if you hit the food refusal stage. It doesn't mean you have a 'fussy eater', and being too quick to label your little ones as such might make the refusal more prolonged.

Instead, think of it as merely a phase and try not to change up what you offer or what you do and serve around the table too much. Some things that have been tried and tested and are backed by research include:

- Avoid pressures to eat up – they actually have the opposite effect.

- Role model eating and enjoying foods.

- Have fun at mealtimes.

- Offer smaller portions, especially of new foods.

- Allow them to eat to appetite and avoid predicting what they need.

- Avoid alternatives and instead suggest another day you can have the requested food.

- Stick to a routine around meals and snacks.

- Offer a wide variety of foods.

- Avoid drawing attention when foods are refused and move on with the meal.

- Look at what your children are eating over a week, not just in a single day or at a single meal.

- Expect variations in appetites.

Focusing the attention around food and food refusal can sometimes be unhelpful. Take the pressures off 'eating' and try to make those meals light and enjoyable together as much as you can.

Making separate meals

Ideally, we want the meals we share together to be as similar as possible, so that our children can start to emulate and copy our own eating behaviours and get familiar with eating the same meals, flavours, tastes and textures as the rest of the family. This makes it much easier going forward when you're creating one meal for everyone to share.

Starting with this early on and getting babies used to home-cooking styles and flavours at the start of weaning can help, as can keeping on trying meals over time – even ones that are less familiar and get refused.

Making separate meals for everyone just isn't practical, and is likely to end up with us as parents/carers cooking a lot extra, spending more time in the kitchen and less time resting or playing with our kids. If we're making separate meals, it's also likely to cost us more, lead to more food waste, and actually encourage more fussy eating/food refusal in the long run.

Instead, there are ways to try to encourage sharing meals and to try to have similar meals, including:

 From a young age, try to build flavours, textures and typical family-style meals into your baby's diet.

 Remember, it's often easy to leave bits of the meal out e.g., honey drizzled on top that isn't suitable for babies, or to forgo the salt in a recipe until the end or chop/grind nuts into a recipe rather than offering them whole.

 It's also often easy to alter the texture of a small portion of the dish, for example mashing a bit more with a fork for a baby or blending parts of the meal if the texture isn't quite right. It doesn't mean they can't have the same meal, it might just need adapting.

 Avoid adding salt and sugar, and instead use extra herbs and spices to add flavour, or simply season your own adult portions at the end.

Offer little table buffets and encourage everyone (aside from babies) to help themselves and build their own plates, regularly.

 Try to bring in something 'familiar' to the meal so that there is always something for young ones to eat.

 Allow new sauces and dishes to be offered on the plate in small amounts, so if it's new curry dish, offer plenty of rice and add some extra veggies and keep the portion of something 'new' small.

 Avoid or limit heavy spices in meals you're sharing and gradually help them build up tolerance for any strong spices used. Other herbs and mild spices are fine to cook with.

 Allow them to pick out bits that they don't like – that's OK, but try not to draw too much attention to it and just focus on eating the whole meal yourself.

 Allow seconds of any part of the meal they do like, if available, and avoid commenting on bits they have left.

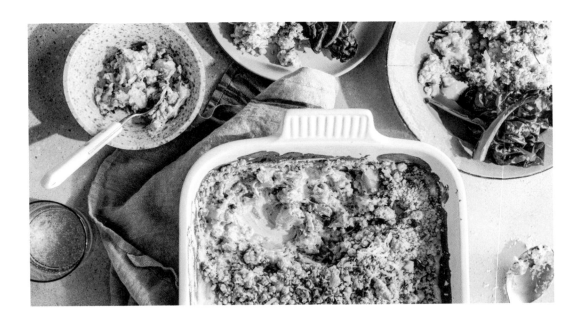

Catering for Allergies

Catering for a child or children with an allergy can be a challenge, and there is no doubt that it will make planning meals and recipes a little more difficult in your household. However, creating fun, exciting, vibrant and healthy meals that the whole family can share is still very much possible.

Here are some of my tips for family meals when you have to cater for one or multiple allergies in your household:

You could completely exclude the allergen/allergens from your home – this can make cooking easier as you know that everything you have in the cupboards is safe to use. However, this might depend on how many allergens your child is allergic to, and how easy you find adapting your meals.

Have some main staple meals that you can all eat that are allergy-friendly and safe for the whole family. Make them in bulk when you can, freeze them, and use them as emergency meal options. I have some recipes in my books, but also Allergy UK has a wealth of resources and recipes online to inspire you and there are multiple websites and cookbooks focused on 'free-from' recipes.

Use substitutions where possible. There are so many look-a-like, accessible and simple substitutes on the market these days so there are plenty to choose from, for example: egg replacers or chia seed eggs, plant-based spreads instead of butter, plant milks instead of dairy, gluten-free pastas and bread, and multiple versions of nut butters, tahini and even a 'no-nuts nut butter' you can get online (see page 108 for more ideas).

Label foods properly and ensure that anything that you've cooked, opened or bought is clearly labelled as an allergen/allergen-free, especially anything you add to the freezer as it's easy to forget.

If you do decide to keep allergens in the home, have a shelf in the fridge and a cupboard that is dedicated to just the allergen-friendly foods and ingredients.

Create a stash of freezer allergen-free snacks. It can be challenging when going to parties, playdates and out with other families if your child is the only one without a snack. Find some snacks your kid loves and make a mountain of them to freeze for a later date.

 Cook from scratch as much as possible – I know it's tough, but it can help you to practise cooking without the allergen and be more in control of what's going into a meal without having to check labels and read up about ingredients. The more familiar you get with allergy-free cooking the better.

 Educate your whole family on how to protect your food-allergic child from their allergen.

 Educate your child and, as soon as they are old enough, teach them to always say no to foods they've been given and to check with an adult before eating them.

 Speak to your child's healthcare professional about the allergy, get details on the severity and the possibility of reintroduction down the line.

 Have an allergy plan for the whole family and for anyone who cares for your child, including school and nursery.

 Keep any allergy kits nearby at all times.

 Become a pro at reading labels and ensure you know exactly what to look out for and what things like 'trace of' or 'made in a factory with' labels mean for your child. If you're unsure, speak to your healthcare professional.

 Understand the rules for safe preparation – put up some kitchen rules for everyone to see whenever food is being prepared in the kitchen and make sure everyone knows and follows these rules at all times.

 Stress the importance of hygiene around mealtimes and put in plans to avoid cross-contamination – you might need separate plates and utensils for your allergy child or just to label things a lot when you are cooking/storing foods.

 Cook your allergy-friendly dishes first to avoid the risk of cross-contamination.

 Cover any foods for your children who are allergic and pop them high up in the fridge to avoid cross-contamination.

3

GETTING
ORGANISED

It can feel so overwhelming thinking about how many meals you need to cook each week, and how to make them healthy, while also trying to ensure everyone is happy and meals get eaten, but without spending your whole life chained to the oven or all weekend organising your fridge.

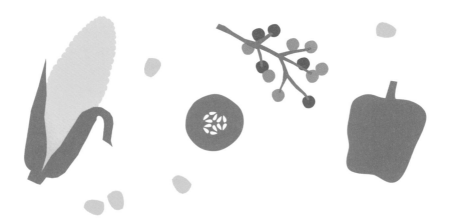

In this chapter I've outlined everything you need to know to make food storage and prep easier, but also to help you reduce food waste, make the most of your kitchen and make creating food more enjoyable and less time-consuming.

You'll see that I've included lots of hacks, tricks and graphics throughout to help you get to the bottom of what you need at a glance – food already takes so much of our headspace! I really hope you find it helpful.

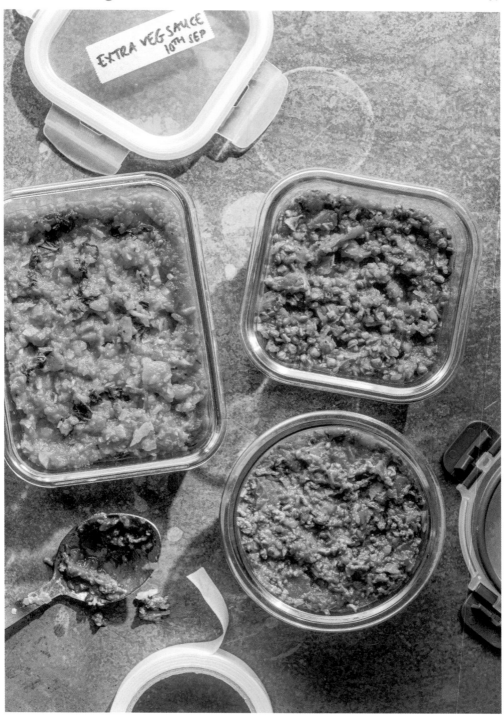

Organising Your Fridge

Stocking your fridge is all about minimising risk to your health by keeping foods edible and safe for as long as possible. This guide is going to give you all the details you need to know about safely and practically packing your fridge.

Keep ready-to-eat foods and leftovers at eye level/at the top of the fridge. These are lower risk but can act as a prompt to remind you to use them.

Eggs should be kept in the fridge, ideally, and in the main body of the fridge, so the shelf above the meats should work fine for these. Do not store eggs in the door as the temperature here is too variable.

The fridge should be between 0–5°C at all times.

Raw meat, poultry and fish needs to be kept low in the fridge because this section has a lower temperature, so put these just above the salad drawers.

Keeping foods low minimises the risk of contamination. Use a separate plate or plastic box to help keep high-risk foods separate.

Store fruit, vegetables and salads in the bottom drawers. This helps keep fresh food safe from contamination, and helps it to last longer.

The bottom of the fridge is the safest place for foods as it has a constant temperature and humidity.

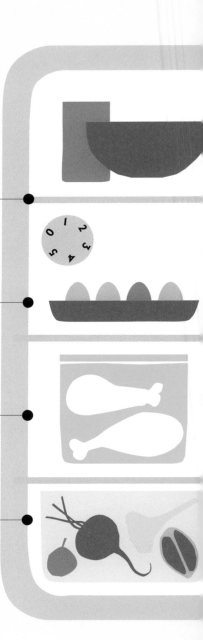

The door should only contain the lowest risk food as it's the most variable temperature of the fridge. Juices and condiments with long shelf lives should stay here.

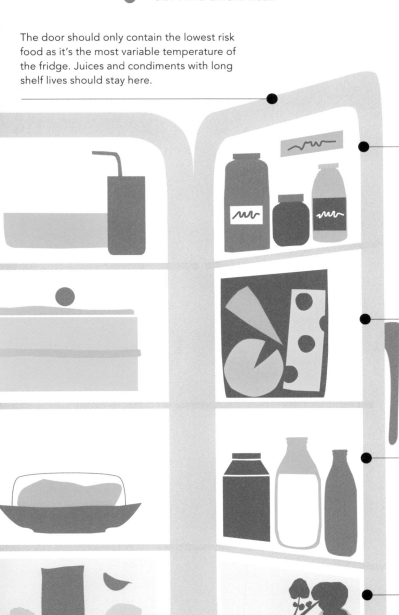

General tips:

Have labels for your fridge so it's clear what dates things were opened/need using by.

Label each shelf so each member of your family knows where everything goes – keep labels and a pen handy; even in your fridge if you can!

Use storage containers, lidded plates and food wrap to keep foods safe before and after cooking.

Clean up any spills immediately and clean your fridge around once a week.

Keep the fridge door open for as short time as possible.

Try not to overstock the fridge.

Keep some cool packs in your fridge/freezer in case of emergencies or even just to throw into lunch bags for on the go.

Chop up veggies and store them in glass Tupperware so they are easy to see and to grab and go.

BEFORE YOU SHOP

MAKE A LIST of things you absolutely need and try not to deviate from this.

KNOW your labels – 'use by' and 'best before' mean different things.

FACTOR IN occasions when you're likely to eat out so whole meals don't go to waste.

BRING OUT FOODS that need using up soon and plan them into a meal for that day.

MAKE A MEAL PLAN! It can save you time, energy and brain space when you know exactly what's being eaten each day.

CHECK THE FRIDGE, cupboards and freezer to make sure you don't buy things you already have.

AVOID shopping when you're hungry.

HOW TO REDUCE

ONCE YOU'RE HOME

DOWNLOAD a smart fridge app or a digital food guide to help you manage and reduce food waste.

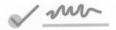

MAKE A LIST (ideally on the front of the fridge) of all the ingredients you need to use up and what you could make them into (see page 66).

TRY TO SAVE SOME TIME to wash, clean and prep any foods that you know you won't use for a while. You can freeze so many foods like berries, milk, cheese and veggies.

ORDER your foods according to what needs using first – put new versions of foods behind old versions or label them.

Check where you need to store foods to ensure they last as long as they should (see page 60).

USE bag clips or bulldog clips to keep foods fresh where possible.

HAVE A 'LEFTOVERS' SHELF in the fridge so you can instantly see what needs using up.

CHECK the fridge temperature – it should be 0–5°C.

WHEN YOU'RE SHOPPING

STICK TO YOUR LIST – it's only really a deal if you actually needed it in the first place. Avoid overbuying as it leads to food waste!

AVOID THE KIDS' 'PESTER POWER' by getting them involved with the shopping and helping you with loading and unloading!

IF YOU'RE SHOPPING ONLINE, create a favourites list and use that each time you log in.

AS YOU'RE GOING AROUND, make a note of foods you'll need to use fairly quickly so you can make some meals with them in the next few days.

FOOD WASTE AT HOME

WHEN COOKING

TRY TO have meals together as a family so you're cooking one meal for everyone.

SWAP DIFFERENT VEGGIES out if you have some that need using up. Most recipes can easily be adapted.

BULK-MAKE MEALS and freeze individual portions so you have control over how much you defrost each time.

MAKE A 'LEFTOVER' soup or sauce that combines foods that need using up. You can bulk-make and freeze (see page 142, Leftover Veg Soup).

SERVE SMALL PORTIONS (especially for picky family members) and allow for seconds so that untouched leftovers can be eaten on another day or frozen.

LABEL DISHES when storing them, with the name of the dish and the date you made it, to ensure you eat it within a safe period of time.

MAKE LEFTOVERS into omelettes, muffins, cakes, soups, stews and sauces.

IF RECIPES call for foods you don't normally use, swap out with an alternative that you already have in your kitchen. See page 108 for alternative food ideas.

Most wasted foods in the UK, and what to do with them when they are on their way out:

BREAD

Blend into breadcrumbs and freeze for a later date. You can make homemade fish fingers, katsu curry or chicken/tofu nuggets.

Chop into squares and fry with a little oil and rosemary to turn into crunchy croutons.

Toast and add chopped garlic and butter to the top to serve as a side.

Dice them up and store them in a bag in the freezer to easily throw into recipes.

ONIONS AND GARLIC

POTATO

Chop any roots/less appealing bits off, then peel. Slice and freeze for layering on top of pies.

Peel, chop, boil and turn into mashed potato – you can also freeze this.

Mash well and add to bakes and cakes in place of sugar or eggs e.g., replace eggs in pancake recipes or sugar in banana bread.

BANANAS

Slice them and freeze them in layers and add to smoothies at a later date.

Slice them (before browning), brush each one with a little lemon juice, olive oil or honey and roast for 20 minutes.

TOMATOES

Turn them into a sauce – see my tomato sauce recipe on page 166, or creamy tomato and spinach gnocchi on page 162. Simply blend or simmer in a pan with some herbs and other veggies, and voila!

MILK Freeze it! Milk freezes pretty well and just needs a little shake or stir on defrosting.

Add it to soups, sauces and béchamel to make your dinner a little creamy.

Dice and freeze it when you get it, if you're not using it right away. **POULTRY**

CARROTS Dice or cut into batons and freeze them for easy options to add to meals or easy finger food options for older kids.

Tear it up, add some chopped tomatoes, drizzle over balsamic vinegar and offer as a side salad with any meal. **LETTUCE**

MOST FRUITS Puree/chop up and freeze to add to porridge or puddings.

Blend into a smoothie with some yoghurt.

Mash and cook with some chia seeds over the hob to make into jam, see page 203.

Chop, then add to soups or dinners as an extra portion of veg. **MOST VEG**

Chop and store in a bag in the freezer for later use in sauces, soups and other dinners.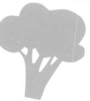

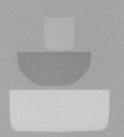

Food to use chart

Use this chart on your fridge and/or freezer to help you keep track of what needs to be used up in the next few days and help you reduce your food waste.

Visit www.srnutrition.co.uk to download your own chart.

FOOD TO USE UP...	USE IT BY?	MAKE IT INTO?
e.g., yoghurt	12/12/23	Offer it at breakfast tomorrow
Carrot	2 days	Dice and add to tonight's dinner
Cheese	1 week	Grate it onto tomorrow's salad

Organising Your Freezer

Using your freezer effectively is a bit of a minefield, but, once you've cracked it, you can be sure that you'll never go back to your old ways. There are so many foods that can be frozen and a much shorter list of foods that don't do so well in the freezer.

Making the most of your freezer can help you meal plan, reduce waste and be more efficient at creating your family meals.

What can't I freeze?

You can actually freeze pretty much anything; it's more about how it comes out of the freezer and whether it still 'works' in your dish. Some foods, such as salads and high-water foods like cucumber, don't freeze well and although they are fine from a 'safe to eat' and nutritional point of view, they will be pretty mushy and unappealing!

Soft cheeses, boiled eggs, mayonnaise and other emulsified foods like cream cheese don't have great textures when frozen and defrosted – eggs go rubbery and mayonnaise/cream cheese separate so can't really be used. Other than that, most things can easily be frozen so try to make the use of your freezer when you can!

Freezing foods and nutrition

Frozen foods get a bad reputation nutritionally, but actually if you freeze foods at their peak freshness, you can lock in a lot of the nutrients in that food. Variety is ideal and using frozen foods/ freezing foods at home is definitely a good option for reducing waste, feeding the family and helping you save time and energy. Plus, it is also unlikely to vastly alter a food's nutritional profile as long as it's not frozen for really long periods of time – the ideal length for most foods is three to six months.

Before you begin to organise your freezer, have a good declutter first and work out how to use up some of the meals and foods you have in there, before starting again from scratch. It does depend on the amount of space and type of freezer you have, so the tips here are general guides for all freezer styles.

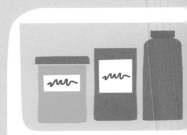

Keep foods you use a lot near the top so you can pop them in and out of the freezer quickly – this saves energy and prevents the freezer from getting iced up.

A full freezer is a more efficient one as it takes less energy to keep everything cool.

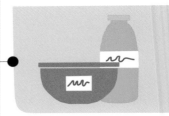

Keep foods that need to be used up first and short expiry date products at the front. Put newer items towards the back/bottom.

Label foods, especially if they are homemade, so you know what they are, when they were frozen and when to use them by.

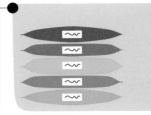

Use freezer bins, boxes or storage file dividers to keep your freezer tidy and to help you see everything more easily.

Have a zone for foods you need to use up soon, if you have the space, or store them where you can see them easily.

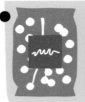

Freeze liquids, fruits and veggies in ziplock bags flat to utilise more space. Once frozen, move them to upright, filing system-style arrangement.

Freeze individual foods like berries or apple slices open (laid out on a baking tray) and then pop into a freezer bag. This helps them to freeze quickly, preserve the quality and stop them clumping together.

When defrosting food from your freezer, pop it in the fridge overnight or run water over the sealed container/bag to loosen the contents slightly before adding to a pan/oven and heating all the way through. You can also use the 'defrost' setting on your microwave.

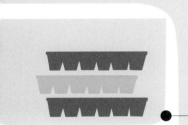

Your freezer should be -18°C at all times.

Ensure you clean it regularly and defrost it once every six months to help it work effectively.

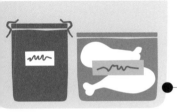

Invest in some good reusable freezer bags and boxes – get them in all shapes and sizes to fit different amounts of food. Use clips and seals effectively to keep products closed and prevent freezer burn.

Freeze foods in realistic portions so that you can defrost the amount that you actually need.

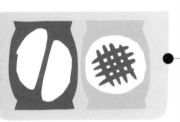

Wrap/seal foods tightly and try to remove any air/ fill containers completely as much as possible before putting them in the freezer. Use a vacuum sealer to help take the air out more easily.

Have a dedicated 'random items' box in the freezer for the little bags of things that don't fit into a specific category, such as breadcrumbs or lime slices.

Organise your freezer by category. Have 'zones' for different products, such as bakery, fruit and veg, or meat and fish. Label shelves/drawers in your freezer.

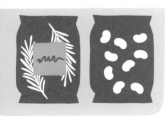

Use baking parchment between individual food items (e.g. pancakes) to stop them freezing together.

Have a freezer inventory or use a wipeable marker pen on the front of your fridge or a magnetic dry-wipe board, to put details of what you need to use up over the next days. Alternatively, use the 'Food to Use' chart on page 66.

Tips for Cooking on a Budget

A lot of the information in this book should help you with cooking and preparing meals for your family on a budget, especially messages on reducing food waste and menu planning. It's important that creating healthy foods for your family doesn't cost you huge amounts and I've created plenty of budget-friendly, store-cupboard staples in the recipe section in this book. Check out the 'alternative ingredients' table on page 108 to help you make some swaps for any ingredients which you struggle to access or are a little more of a stretch on your meal-planning budget.

I've shared lots of tips below to help with your food-shop budgeting – I hope you find this helpful!

- Visit the supermarket at the end of the day if you can, when fresh foods are often on offer. You can freeze anything that you can't use immediately. Chop up herbs, veggies or fruits, and blend tomatoes, before freezing them.
- Shop around. Spend some time initially finding out where you can buy cheaper food group items, such as fruits and veg, grains in bulk, and meat and fish. Sometimes you'll be surprised by how cheap they can be from local shops instead of supermarkets.
- Try to make an effort to buy plenty of ingredients in bulk as it's much cheaper. Pasta, grains, oats, dried lentils and beans, and herbs and spices are all good options to buy in bulk as they last and can come out much cheaper in larger amounts.
- Buy batches of foods such as meat, fruit and veg that are on their last legs at the supermarket, then chop and freeze them.
- Buy foods like onions and potatoes that are close to their best before date when you're doing a big batch-cook day, use it all quickly and add it to your freezer stash.
- Use less meat in recipes as meat is expensive, and bulk it out with cheaper ingredients such as dried or tinned beans.
- Use frozen foods. There are so many frozen veggies and fruits now, and frozen fish and meats are also really handy.

Buy foods in season, as they are are often cheaper than out of season.

Use 'wonky veg' – some schemes do deliveries of wonky veg and some supermarkets offer cheap boxes of veg that are slightly wonky. This can save you a huge amount of money!

Make the most of discount cards from the supermarket or any food vouchers.

Check the global foods aisle when shopping at the supermarket. Sometimes you can buy bulk packets or get products cheaper there.

Don't be afraid of own-brand products – often they contain similar ingredients and are sometimes even made in the same factories as more expensive brands.

Visit the 'discount' stand at the supermarket or even in your greengrocers – often they have foods that are about to go past their best on sale. If you can, freeze or use up as soon as possible.

Stick to your list! Some people find writing a list of what they don't need helps, especially if they're in the habit of buying extras of certain ingredients (we do it with kidney beans and chickpeas every time!).

Grow your own! So many things including chives, mint, parsley, cress and even carrots and strawberries are easy to grow at home, even without a garden.

Plan fridge-raid meals. Once a week try to have a fridge-raid meal where you just check the fridge and use up anything leftover in one big buffet. You'll be surprised at how 'balanced' this can be.

Plan it all out. Meal planning can help you save money by reducing food waste and limiting overbuying. It can also help you prep fewer meals as you can factor in leftovers and leftover ingredients.

Use all the bits of meat when cooking to make one meal go further. For example, after a roast, use the carcass to make a bone broth, which you can use in soups.

BROCCOLI AND CELERY
Wrap in foil, which helps
to keep it fresher for
longer.

SPINACH AND OTHER LEAVES
Put in an airtight container lined
with kitchen paper (this helps
to soak up the extra moisture).
Or line your salad drawer with
paper towels and add your
leaves to this directly.

CARROTS Wrap up in wet
paper towels and put in a
ziplock bag in the fridge (I
use reusable ziplock bags
and clean and reuse again).

HACKS FOR MAKING

LIMES Slice and freeze or
pop in the fridge in a bag.

CUCUMBERS Store
in a cool space in a
compostable bag
with holes in it on
the kitchen counter,
not in the fridge.

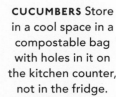

**KIWI, APPLES AND
PEARS** Keep them
separate as they release
a gas that makes them
ripen faster!

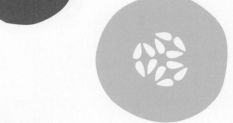

POTATOES, ONIONS AND GARLIC
Store in a cool, dark space, not
in the fridge. Store apples with
potatoes as the ethylene (released
from apples) should make the
potatoes last longer.

BANANAS Wrap the top in cling
film (or beeswax paper) and
store away from other foods.

SPRING ONIONS AND ASPARAGUS Store in a glass of water in the fridge with a loose covering of their wrapping over the top.

FRESH HERBS Keep in a glass of water in the fridge with a loose covering of their wrapping over the top, or wrapped in a wet paper towel in a ziplock bag in the fridge. If you're using herbs a lot, chop and add to an ice cube tray along with some olive oil for use in your cooking.

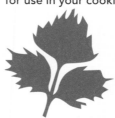

PEPPERS Keep in a bag (I use compostable bags) with holes in it in the fridge.

FOOD LAST LONGER

BLUEBERRIES, STRAWBERRIES AND OTHER BERRIES Soak in water with a few splashes of vinegar added for a few minutes (it doesn't alter the taste of the berries), then drain and pop in an airtight container lined with kitchen paper.

HOMEMADE SAUCES LIKE HUMMUS AND PESTO Cover the top of these with a layer of olive oil to help keep them fresh for longer.

AVOCADO Once cut open, rub lemon or lime juice on the exposed flesh to stop it browning.

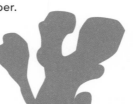

FRESH GINGER Keep in the freezer – it's easier to grate and peel and lasts a long time.

OTHER TIPS:

Use vacuum seals on your storage containers if you have them.

Use an 'ethylene-absorbing disc' in your fridge to help keep food fresher for longer.

Tips for Menu Planning

If you feel your organisational skills are up to it, menu planning can be such a help. Menu planning can help you prepare, balance your meals for your family, reduce food waste, eat more varied meals, experiment more, have more fun with ingredients, take everyone's tastes into account… and so much more. In fact, while writing this book, I started to do a lot more menu planning and it really saved us time and money, so it's well worth a go. Here are some of my tips on making it work:

- Have a blank, glass A4 photo frame in the kitchen and write out your meals for the week on it using a washable marker (you can also use apps on your phone too if you're more technically savvy!).

- Get everyone in the family on board and get them to vote for their favourite meals to go on the menu each week.

- Have recipes/meal ideas written up on cards so you have inspiration at your fingertips when putting the menu plan together. Keep the cards all together in your kitchen so you have a constant supply of inspiration.

- Before you start the meal plan, take a look at what's in the fridge and freezer so you can first use up things you already have.

- Have theme nights once a week or once a month to help you experiment with new recipes. These can include Mexican nights, soup nights or 'leftover' nights.

- Regularly add your family's favourite meals into the meal plans so that everyone gets a turn eating something they love!

- Double up recipes you're cooking regularly and freeze them for busier days in the week – add these frozen meals to your menu plan so you don't forget about them. Remember to label them with the date made and what it is.

Once a week or month (family situation dependent) have a 'freezer meal' where you use a ready meal or a frozen meal you've made before to save you time. Simply defrost in the fridge overnight and heat thoroughly before you eat!

Don't be afraid of subbing ingredients when your plan doesn't quite work. Nothing works out exactly how we want it to, and it's very easy to swap different veggies, carbs or flavours into meals (see page 108 for more on this).

Have some 'emergency' options at your disposal if and when you need them. Store-cupboard staples (see page 96) are always a winner in my house: pasta and sauce, beans on toast, frozen veg with couscous or good old porridge can always work for those emergency meals.

The meal planner overleaf is a great example of a balanced mealplan and how to prep meals. For more on this and blank templates, visit **www.srnutrition.co.uk** to download your own.

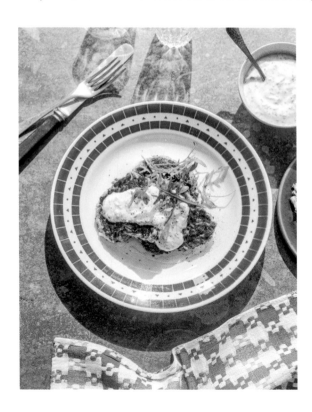

	BREAKFAST	LUNCH
SUNDAY	Fluffy Coconut Pancakes (p. 122) **10–20 mins prep** Freeze leftovers OR Easy Family Smoothie (p. 111) **5 mins prep**	Tuna Orzo Salad (p. 135) **15 mins prep** Start prep Pork Casserole (p. 174) for dinner **5 mins prep**
MONDAY	Baked Banana Bars (from yesterday) with glass of milk	Stuffed Calzone Pittas (p.143) **10 mins prep**
TUESDAY	Porridge/usual cereal with toppings, e.g.- mixed fruits, seeds, nut butter Bake leftovers into porridge muffins (+ oats/ banana + bake for 20mins. Freeze extras or use as snacks)	Dinner Leftovers (Veg & Lentil Pie) OR Quick Veggie Frittata (p. 129) **20 mins prep**
WEDNESDAY	Apple Crumble Bircher Freeze any leftovers or use as a snack. Take Dahl out of freezer for dinner – pop in fridge	Salmon Paté (or hummus) on Toast (p. 132) **5 mins prep**
THURSDAY	Porridge/usual cereal – add mixed fruits, etc. Bake leftovers into porridge muffins (+ oats/ banana + bake for 20mins. Freeze extras or use as snacks) Take dinner out of freezer, if using	Sandwiches + fillings (e.g. Egg & Avocado Hummus & Red Pepper Smoked Salmon & Cream Cheese Tomato & Mozzarella)
FRIDAY	Toast topping - e.g. Smashed Avocado & Chive or scrambled egg (p. 118)	Cheesy Greens Pasta (p. 140) **10 mins prep**
SATURDAY	Blueberry Breakfast Muffins Make a batch & freeze leftovers Start prep for Comforting Chicken Soup (p. 138) for lunch	Comforting Chicken Soup OR Mexican Tomato Soup (p. 160) **20 mins prep**

DINNER	SNACK	PREP
Pork Casserole OR Leftover Veg Soup (p. 142) **10 mins prep** Freeze any leftovers for next week	Oat cakes/crackers with dip + veg sticks (shop-bought or recipes in this book, p. 201)	**Make 1–2 hours today to batch cook:** Sweet Potato & Lentil Dahl (p. 152) **15 mins prep** Oaty Cookie (p. 212) **10 mins prep** Baked Banana Bars (p. 120) **5 mins prep** (save some for Monday) Freeze all
Green Veg & Lentil Pie (p. 155) **10 mins prep**	Rice cakes or toast with nut butter (p. 219) + veg sticks	Take oaty cookies out of freezer & pop in fridge for tomorrow's snack
Baked Risotto (p. 168) **10 mins prep**	Oaty Cookie (from fridge) + fruit slices	Make ahead Apple Crumble Bircher Muesli (p. 112) for tomorrow's breakfast **5 mins prep** Get Banana Bars out of freezer. Pop in fridge to defrost
Freezer meal: E.g. Sweet Potato & Lentil Dahl from Sunday's prep	Baked Banana Bars (from freezer or leftovers) with a dip	**In the AM** – Get dinner out of the freezer for this evening's meal
Use leftover freezer meal from Sunday e.g. Pork Casserole OR Leftover Veg Soup OR Pad Thai (p.170) **10 mins prep**	Porridge muffin with yogurt + nut butter dip.	**In the AM** – Get dinner meal out of the freezer for this evening's meal Make ahead Carrot, Date & Coconut Energy Balls (p. 202) **5 mins prep**
Quorn Fajitas (p. 156) **10–20 mins prep**	Small portion of leftover meals/snacks from the week e.g. bircher, pancakes, energy balls	**In the AM** – Take out snacks from freezer for today Make ahead Blueberry Breakfast Muffins (p. 114) for next day breakfast **5–10 mins prep**
Cheat's Veggie Lasagne (p. 178) Freeze leftovers for next week. **20 mins prep**	Carrot, Date & Coconut Energy Balls made midweek, or mini sandwiches and fillings	

Tips for Batch Cooking

Let's face it, batch cooking can really help but you need to have the time to do it. I try to find a period when I have time to myself (usually Saturday mornings when the kids all go out for football) and I put on my favourite music or a podcast and get cooking. Having two hours to batch cook like this makes a massive difference to my whole week. It means I have meals, snacks and random food options at the ready throughout the week without having to think about it too much. Try to include these batch-cooked meals in your weekly meal plan and remember to label foods and use the little toolkits I've included to help you keep your fridge and freezer foods at the front of your mind.

Here are some tips on batch cooking efficiently:

Give yourself time – make sure you aren't rushing, as this can end in disaster.

It feels like there's always more important things to do, but batch cooking can help you have more time in the week, so prioritise it where you can.

Create some space before you start!

Start with a clean kitchen and an empty dishwasher to make the clean-up much simpler.

Plan ahead – make sure you have the ingredients you need and space in your fridge or freezer. It helps if your cupboards and fridge are organised too.

You don't need special equipment but large pans, soup makers or slow cookers, various sizes of storage containers, freezer bags and labels are all super handy.

Prep all the ingredients first. This allows you to follow the recipe much more smoothly.

Make it enjoyable – listen to a podcast or do it over a glass of wine (perhaps not on a Saturday morning!) or play some music.
It really cheers me up when I do this.

Cool all foods before freezing. A cold water bath (once foods are sealed and ready to freeze) can do this.

Bunging ingredients into a slow cooker while you sort out a different recipe can be a godsend. They aren't often expensive but can be very handy if you're planning on bulk cooking a lot.

Choose some recipes that can make multiple meals throughout the week. For example, tomato sauce with can be used as a base for a chilli, lasagne, pasta sauce, stew, curry or a jacket potato topping.

Avoid over-seasoning, as the flavours in the food may be enhanced over time, and it's hard to remember how much you've already used. You can always season at the table if you need to.

Get your ingredients and equipment out ready before you begin. Creating recipes over the last few years for my books, I've found that this really cuts the 'hands-on' time down when you're cooking.

Choose super simple meals to batch cook and pop them in the freezer. I like to have an 'emergency' tomato sauce in the freezer at all times.

Clear up as you go along – pop ingredients back in the cupboard and put any equipment you've used straight in the dishwasher or sink.

Choosing some super simple options means you have more meals you can make in your allocated time.

Make a recipe such as banana bread or flapjacks that you know will last your family the week, so you have a 'go-to' snack options.

Don't forget to slice anything before you freeze it so it's easy to take out just one portion.

Be realistic with time. Leave 30 mins–1 hour for each recipe end to end, and if you have more time, it's a bonus!

If you've got a lot of chopping to do, a box vegetable chopper or a food processor can do the hard jobs for you.

You can easily add 'extras' later – stirring in yoghurt, adding lentils or a tin of kidney beans – all with minimum effort!

Shopping list

Below is a shopping list template ordered by supermarket aisles so you can do your shopping in order! Download your copy at **www.srnutrition.co.uk**

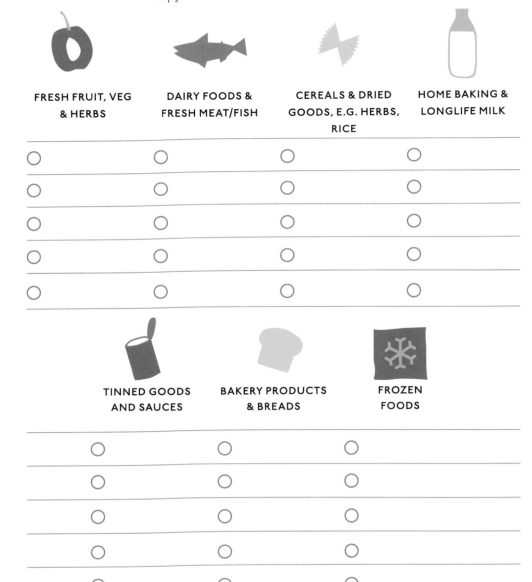

FRESH FRUIT, VEG & HERBS   DAIRY FOODS & FRESH MEAT/FISH   CEREALS & DRIED GOODS, E.G. HERBS, RICE   HOME BAKING & LONGLIFE MILK

TINNED GOODS AND SAUCES   BAKERY PRODUCTS & BREADS   FROZEN FOODS

Preparing Food Safely

When you're prepping foods for the family, it's important to follow standard food safety guidelines and to be aware of some of the foods that might pose more of a risk of food poisoning as children have less well-developed immune systems than adults.

From a food hygiene and safety perspective, some of the key things you need to know about handling foods in the kitchen include:

- **Wash hands before cooking** as well as after and between prepping different foods.
- **Wash cutting boards** and any kitchen equipment after handling raw meat and fish.
- Use **different chopping boards for different food stuffs**, especially if you're prepping raw meat and fish.
- **Wash fruits and veggies** well before prepping them to eat.
- **Defrost food in your fridge** (not at room temperature) so it defrosts at a lower temperature.
- **Cook foods thoroughly.** Don't be tempted to only reheat a little so it's not too hot for little ones – reheat it fully, until piping hot, then let it cool.
- **Cook meat and fish well**, all the way through.

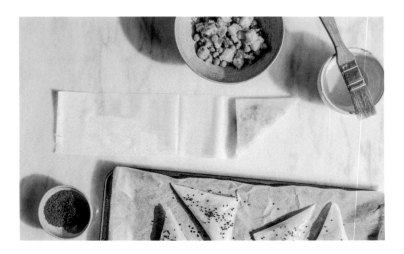

There are also some foods you need to be mindful of not offering to young children, or limiting or adapting so that they become safer for them to eat. Even into the toddler years (and certainly as babies) there are some foods that are more likely to pose a choking risk.

Be careful of foods that are:

- hard and break off in chunks
- hard and round
- round and squidgy with soft edges
- hard to chew
- slippery

These can all pose a choking risk to small children. As toddlers hone their eating skills they will be more able to cope with these foods, but you can always easily prep them until then by chopping, cooking, squashing or grating, for example.

Guidelines for a lot of these foods are not to offer them until around four to five years of age, but it does vary.

Notice how your child's eating skills develop and how well they cope with certain textures of foods. Some children will have adult-style eating earlier than others, but four to five years of age is a good estimation of when they are likely to have fully developed oral motor skills in place (for example, using their teeth well and moving foods around in their mouth easily, as well as being able to spit out anything they need to). Make sure you are always with them when they eat, ensuring they are in a supportive chair and sitting upright, and able to move their arms and hands effectively.

You can be mindful of these foods while still offering some safely, depending on your little one's ages and skillset. Throughout the recipe section of this book, I've included tips and hacks to help you prep foods for younger babies and toddlers, where needed.

GENERALLY, FOODS TO AVOID/LIMIT OR ADAPT INCLUDE:

WHOLE GRAPES: quarter them lengthways for young children as these can be a choking hazard.

WHOLE NUTS: grind them finely or offer as nut butters for younger babies and toddlers, but for older toddlers with good eating skills well-chopped nuts should be OK. Whole nuts are a choking hazard.

LARGE BLUEBERRIES: give them a little squish with your fingers or chop them up until your little one is a more confident eater.

RAW CARROT AND APPLE: hard chunks of apple and carrot can be a risk for choking as big chunks can easily break off and get lodged in the windpipe. Offer these foods grated, mashed or well-cooked and sliced into sticks until your toddler has good eating skills.

SAUSAGES: offer these sliced lengthways through the middle, twice.

LARGE SEEDS: these can be a choking hazard. Simply offer ground or chop well before stirring into baby's foods.

LARGE BEANS: offer them sliced, mashed or squashed to younger babies and toddlers.

CHERRY TOMATOES: these can be a choking hazard when served whole. Choose soft varieties, crush them before offering or chop them lengthways in quarters for babies and toddlers. You can also offer larger tomatoes sliced or add them to a sauce.

WHOLE LARGE DRIED FRUITS: these should be offered when babies are older, and even then should be well-chopped. You can also soak them before adding them to young toddler's foods so they are softer and easier to manage.

CHUNKS OF CHEESE: especially for younger children with less of a 'bite', grate or thinly slice for younger toddlers and babies.

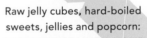

Raw jelly cubes, hard-boiled sweets, jellies and popcorn: **AVOID THESE UNTIL YOUR CHILDREN ARE OLDER.**

Additionally, chop off any really tough bits of food and remove pips and stringy bits for younger children to minimise the risk of choking.

To minimise the risk of choking make sure your baby, toddler or child is:

Sitting in an upright, comfortable position with the ability to easily move their hands and self-feed.

Not alone, someone is always with them when they are eating.

Other foods to be careful with for young babies and toddlers (generally until they are around five years of age):

- Avoid unpasteurised foods like milk and cheese for young children unless well-cooked first.

- Avoid adding salt and sugar to baby's foods (small amounts are inevitable, but try to keep it to a minimum).

- Avoid honey in baby's food before 12 months of age.

- Avoid soft mould-ripened and blue-veined cheeses for young children unless well-cooked first.

- Ensure eggs are well cooked unless they are British Lion Stamped.

- Avoid rice drinks for babies and young children until they are five years of age.

- Limit intakes of oily fish to around two portions for girls and four portions for boys a week.

- Avoid shark, swordfish and marlin for babies and young children. And avoid raw fish, meat and shellfish.

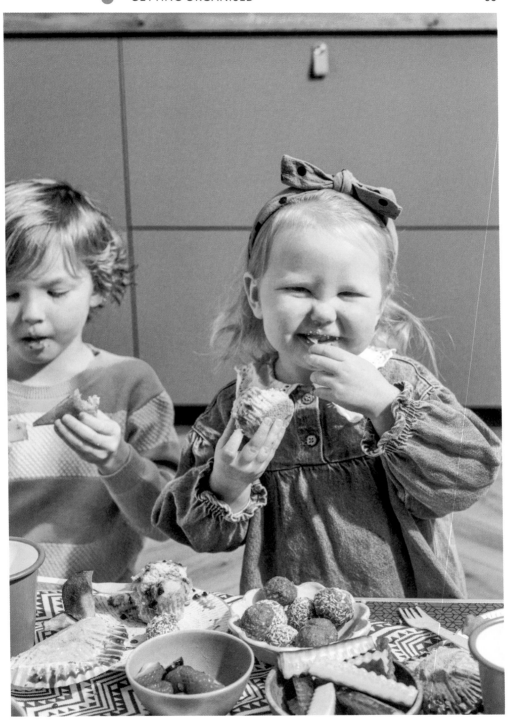

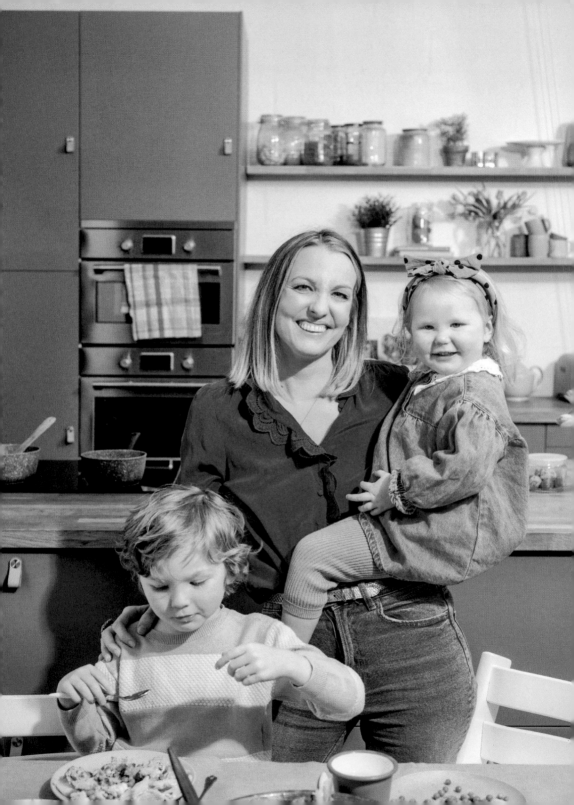

Be Label Savvy

It can be such a challenge understanding food labels – it feels like they are meant to confuse us! Don't pay too much attention to 'halo' claims – 'super food', '1 of your 5 a day', 'contains wholegrains' for example – they can still be a 'less healthy' option. These claims are there to try to encourage you to buy their product, but they don't give you the full picture of what you'll be eating. Here is how to go about checking the nutrition on those labels, for yourself and for your family.

Check the nutritional panel on the packet – it should look something like this:

NUTRITIONAL INFORMATION

Servings per package – 5.5
Serving size – 30g (2/3 cups)

	Per serve	Per 100g
Energy	432k/103Kcal	1441kj/344kcal
Protein	2.8g	9.39g
Fat		
Total	0.4g	1.2g
Saturated	0.1g	0.3g
Carbohydrate		
Total	18.9g	62.9g
Sugars	3.5g	11.8g
Fibre	6.6g	21.2g
Sodium	65mg	215mg

A: check serving sizes that are recommended (a whole packet isn't necessarily one serving).

B: Check levels of salt, sugar and saturated fat. You can check per 100g, which gives you an idea of the % of that product that is sugar, for example, or you can check per serving size, which gives you an idea of how many grams of sugar you'll eat if you eat a serving.

The total sugar content on the nutritional panel includes both added and natural sugars, so the ingredients list can help you work out where sugars (as well as salt) are coming from.

Sugars are usually labelled as '–ose' – for example, glucose, fructose and sucrose – but you may see added sugars appear as 'honey', 'syrups' and 'fruit juice'.

C: Try to choose products with more fibre, vitamins, minerals and protein, and less salt, sugar and saturated fat. If there are any added nutrients, they will likely be listed at the bottom of the panel.

Some questions to ask yourself when looking at the ingredients list:

- Would I expect those ingredients in this product?
- Are sugars and/or salt/salty foods (such as soy sauce, fish sauce or stock) fairly high up in the ingredients list? If so, this means they make up a larger proportion of the product.

INGREDIENTS

Rice, Sugar, Glucose Syrup, Fat Reduced Cocoa Powder, Salt, Cocoa Mass, **Barley** Malt Extract, Flavourings

- Are there some natural/whole foods, such as chunks of apples, banana, dried fruits or even nuts, peanut butter, cheese that might be making the product higher in sugars, fats and salt? If so, these are nutritionally dense foods, so nothing to worry about, but they may make the product higher in sugars, fats and salt.

Just remember that our nutritional intakes and health isn't defined by one food item; it's about what we eat most of the time, regularly and the variety we eat, so don't get stuck on labels – this is just a handy tool to help you understand them better!

Prepping Lunch Boxes for the Family

1. Start with a carbohydrate to offer energy
(ideally wholemeal/wholegrain where possible)

For example:
crackers/oatcakes
stuffed pinwheels
filled sandwiches
pasta salads
wraps
veggie muffins
pitta pizzas
couscous salad
breadsticks for a dip
homemade cheese straws
egg-fried rice
potato salad

Vary the bread: use baps, bagels, chapatti,
sliced bread, wraps, English muffins and pittas
instead of just sliced bread!

2. Add a vegetable (always) and some fruit

For example:
veggie fritters
veggie pancakes
veggie frittata
veggie sticks for a dip
vegetable soup in a flask
veggie muffins
salads in a sandwich or pitta
veggie pizza topping
½ an avocado and a spoon
veggie quiches
whole fruit pieces
sticks of fruit and dip
box of tinned fruits
fruits in yoghurt
fruit skewers
chopped fruit salad box

Try to chop/prep these so they
are easy to eat, where possible.

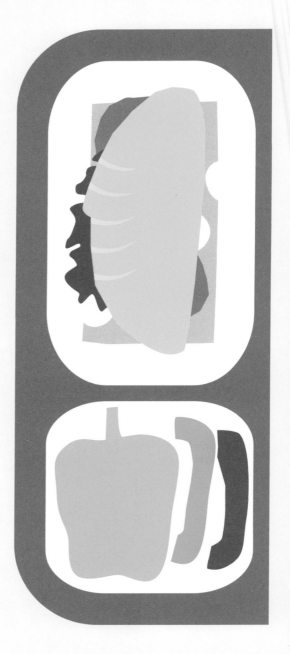

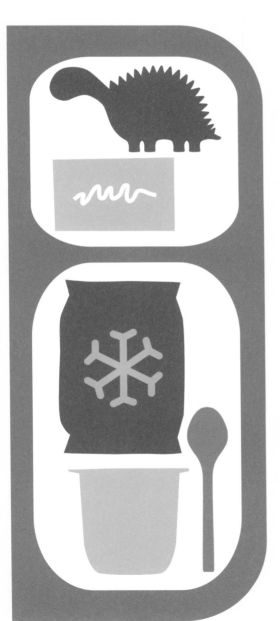

3. Add a protein and a little dairy/alternative

For example:
a carton of milk
a tub of yoghurt
grated cheese in a sandwich/on a pizza
tofu in a wrap
lentils in a soup/pasta sauce
mixed bean salad
shredded chicken
dips e.g., hummus, tahini
tuna salad with couscous
tuna and yoghurt sandwich
hard-boiled egg
fritter/frittata/quiche
chicken soup in a flask
egg-fried rice

Keep these cool with an ice pack
or two in your lunch box.

4. Add something extra for the kids

For example:
cutlery
a napkin
an ice pack
a little note
a small toy

This can help your little ones get a little more excited when it comes to lunchtimes.

5. Add some water in a bottle/flask (freeze it and add instead of an ice pack)

Tips for family lunch boxes

- **Slice and chop foods** so they are easier to eat. A squeeze of lemon can stop fruits and avocado browning and a drizzle of olive oil can help sauces and dips from going hard.

- Have a 'build your own' element for the kids – get them to top their pizzas, mix their sauces, build their own fajita or sprinkle fruit into their yoghurt.

- **Vary** what you offer so lunches don't get too boring!

- Always add a **portion of veggies**.

- **Think outside** of the bread box!

- **Don't forget** about tinned and frozen options too.

- Give kids a **choice** of what goes in or get them to help you with the prep.

- Add a **favourite food** each time so you know something will get eaten.

- Have a **variety of little food boxes** and containers to make it easier to pack different options.

- Use **colourful cupcake cases** to separate foods, if needed.

- **Offer mini food options** such as mini kiwis, cucumbers and peppers for a bit of a novelty factor.

- Use **leftovers** that can be eaten cold for lunch boxes to save you time.

- **Have some bits in your freezer** that make great lunches for lunch boxes in a rush, for example, pinwheels, muffins or pizzas.

- Try to **add lunch-box prep onto other meal prep** so it doesn't take so long.

- **Invest in a good flask and cool packs** to keep foods warm or cool.

- **Use your meal plan** and make sure you're including lunch boxes in it to give you ideas.

- Offer a **'main' and some 'sides' in their lunch box** so it's easy to balance out.

- When choosing a lunch box, you ideally want something that is **spacious, adaptable, fun** for the kids and with plenty of 'areas' for extras such as cutlery or a bottle of water or an ice pack.

Ingredients

Herbs and spices

Some herbs and spices are everyday staples in my house, because they easily add flavour, and bring out so many other flavours in the meal, which means that you really don't need to use salt. Play around with which herbs and spices work for you and your family's tastes.

There are some recipes in this book which use saltier ingredients with the adults in mind (such as soy sauce), but it's still minimal as I really don't feel that foods need a lot of salt if you tap into the delicious flavours coming from herbs and spices.

It's best to avoid offering salt for as long as possible as it's not necessary and it may encourage more of a preference for salty food.

Even from around six months of age when your baby is having their first tastes of foods, you can start to gradually bring in herbs and spices for them to get used to in your home cooking.

Start small with new herbs and do experiment – there is so much you can do once you and your family start really exploring different flavours.

Oils

I've done the research to help us get to the bottom of using oils. In reality, oils vary in their nutritional composition, stability and taste, and uses depending on such a large number of factors: where they are produced, how they are processed, what oils are combined to make your 'vegetable oil', how they are stored, how old they are and how you cook with them. The main thing to remember is that we should include more monounsaturated and polyunsaturated fats in our diet, and less saturated fats. Ultimately if you're using oils:

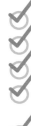

Opt for a variety of oils to use at home.

Choose them for their accessibility, flavour and ease of use.

Avoid overheating oils (don't let them smoke).

Don't heat any oil more than once – they'll start to taste bitter and produce less healthful compounds.

Measure them where you can, to avoid adding too much excess oil.

When frying, use some tissue paper to blot off oil before serving.

NUTMEG: use to bring out the sweetness and add a soft, warm flavour to foods
Add to coffee and hot chocolates
Use in dishes with sweet potato, pumpkin or squash
Stir into butter before adding to potatoes or add to mashed potato for extra creaminess
Add to puddings such as custard, rice pudding or bread puddings
Use in baking such as gingerbreads, biscuits or muffins

CUMIN: an all-rounder with a really warm and earthy flavour
Use in curries, soups and stews to add a really deep flavour
Use in fajita-style dishes or in sauces and marinades
Also works well in burgers and bean burgers
Great for dhal and lentil dishes

HERBS AND

MINT: cooling, but with strong garden vibes
Lovely when made into a tea (and for mojitos!)
Great chopped finely in yoghurt to make a mint-style sauce
Add to puddings which include chocolate, or use as a garnish
Works well with lamb in burgers or roast
Pairs well with peas and asparagus

MIXED HERBS: Always a winner when you're mid-recipe and not sure what to add for flavour!

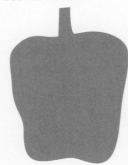

PAPRIKA: adds a sweet kick and a bit of a punch to foods
Add to hummus and dips
Use in stews and soups to add a real depth of flavour
Add to marinades and sauces like harissa to stir into veggies
Sprinkle on hard-boiled eggs or scrambled eggs
Add to rice dishes like risotto or eggy rice
Use as a replacement for hotter spices when cooking for kids

THYME: easy and versatile with a really strong herby, woody flavour
Use with roasted meat, fish and vegetables
Add to dishes where you need plenty of flavour, such as marinades and soups
Perfect in pasta and pizza sauces
Use to garnish recipes or throw in at the end of roasting
Great with mushrooms in a dish and works well with lemon and fish

CINNAMON: use in puddings to add a sweet, nutty, warm kick
Add to the top of cereal and porridge
Sprinkle on yoghurt
Use in home baking
Use on eggy bread
Use in puddings and crumbles

OREGANO: earthy flavour and great in Med-style recipes
Great for pizza and pasta sauces and Italian cooking
Perfect for fresh salads such as Greek salad or with a delicious salad dressing
Great with chicken, fish and bean dishes
Sprinkle over chips and roasted veggies

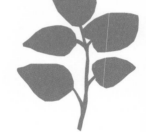

SPICES

CHILLI AND HOT SPICES LIKE CAYENNE:
OK to offer to babies and toddlers, but ideally once they are a little more accustomed to foods
Start small and build up to them, and avoid overdoing it as you may put them off foods

ROSEMARY: a really herby, slightly medicinal flavour
Best for roast potatoes and homemade chips
Also great in roasted vegetable or fish traybakes
Great with garlic, on garlic bread or in focaccia-style breads
Great in soups and casseroles
Good with roasted meats and for use in roast dinners

BASIL: a really fresh, peppery taste
Brilliant with tomatoes or tomato dishes so works with pasta and pizza sauces
Great for turning into sauces such as pesto as it adds lots of flavour
Works well in salads with mozzarella or Parmesan and olive oils
Delicious with new potatoes

PALM OIL

High in saturated and unsaturated fats so less heart-healthy than others

Sustainability issues as palm and soya bean oil make up half of all oils consumed across the world

Cheapest oil and really versatile, hence its use in so many products from shampoo to spreads

OLIVE OIL

High in 'healthy' monounsaturated fatty acids. Extra-virgin olive oil (EVOO) contains higher polyphenols and vitamin E as it is less 'refined', but it's also less versatile as a result. Olive oil has a mild flavour but EVOO has more of a bold, fruity flavour

Olive oil is good for regular cooking at home, frying food, stir-frying and baking. EVOO is less stable, but still OK for general cooking and pan temperatures you reach at home

EVOO is great for salads and consuming cold

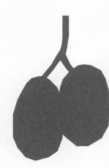

OILS

SOYA BEAN OIL

High in polyunsaturated fatty acids and low in saturated fats

Great for use in salads and as a cooking oil for baking and frying. Quite versatile in day-to-day cooking. Used in spreads a lot

Sustainability issues as it's the most widely used oil in the world, not all for human foods

PEANUT OIL

Contains 'healthy' monounsaturated fats and some polyunsaturated fats and some saturated

Subtle nutty flavour making it great for stir-fry dishes and anything that needs to cook quickly

Used in Chinese and Indian dishes a lot – can be used for deep-fat frying too

Not one of the oils used a great deal in the UK but its use seems to be becoming more popular as 'speciality oils' take off

FLAXSEED OIL

Lots of potential health properties due to high levels of polyunsaturated fatty acid and omega-3 fatty acids.
Source of vitamin E

Shouldn't be used for cooking much as it is very unstable when heated. Use in salads, salad dressings or drizzled over cold dishes

Also called linseed oil

RAPESEED OIL

High in 'healthy' monounsaturated fatty acids (lower in saturated fats than all other vegetable oils). Contains some vitamin E

Super versatile so good for pan-frying at home, general day-to-day cooking and baking

Generically called 'vegetable oil' in the UK – usually it's rapeseed oil

SUNFLOWER OIL

High in polyunsaturated fatty acids (low in saturates)

Different varieties are available, but generally it's good for pan-frying at home and use in general cooking and salad dressings

Used in spreads a lot

WALNUT OIL

Small quantities of saturated fats and mainly polyunsaturated fatty acids present

Contains some beneficial omega-3 fatty acids

Best used on salads, salad dressings and on cold dishes or splashed on soups just before eating

SESAME OIL

Largely 'healthy' poly- and monounsaturated fatty acids, so a positive fatty acid profile. Contains some antioxidants, but varies depending on levels of refining

Used for frying and can reach high temperatures easily

COCONUT OIL

High in saturated fats

Great for use in cooking every now and then, and can be used at high temperatures

Recently has become more popular due to 'purported' health benefits, that aren't founded in research

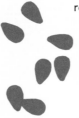

Store-cupboard Staples

There are a few items that I always have in my cupboards and that work as really great options when you need an emergency meal (this happens a lot in our house!). Having these means that you always have a few easy meal options up your sleeve, whatever the weather! Having a balanced meal (see page 16) only takes a few simple ingredients sometimes.

Here are some of my favourite store-cupboard staples and how I use them.

CARBOHYDRATE STAPLES	**Rice** (pre-cooked packets or big bags of dried): easy for a very quick dinner or to add to a curry (see page 158)

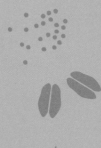

Couscous: a super-quick carb option. Great to add to salads or just simply mix with roasted veggies and a little cheese

Pasta: for pesto pasta (of course!), or to add to soups and stews

Oats: for making a quick pudding with leftover fruit, breakfast in the morning or add to yoghurt as a snack

Potatoes: great for roasting, boiling or just having as an extra side. You can make them into chips, mash or just whack them into a sauce to make a more balanced meal. Jacket potato is always a win too

Crackers: always a good out-and-about option. Great with a spread or a dip

Bread (in the freezer): for beans on toast, to dip into a soup or to have as toast with other toppings (see page 118)

PROTEIN-/IRON-RICH STAPLES

Tinned and frozen fish: add to toast toppings, mix with yoghurt and grains to make a lunch, steam and add to some pasta sauce

Dried and tinned lentils: throw into pasta sauce, pizza toppings or add to soups and stews

Tins of kidney beans and chickpeas: use in curries or chillies or add to salads with a little dressing

Eggs: cook and serve on toast or as eggy bread. Offer hard-boiled as a snack or make into egg-fried rice. Use in baking too

Baked beans: serve on toast or on the side of a meal (such as fish and chips)

Milled flaxseeds (in the fridge): sprinkle on porridge, scatter in salads or use in baking

FRUITS AND VEGGIES

Peas: my favourite side dish, ever! Add to curries, pasta sauces or just enjoy as a snack

Frozen mixed veggies: throw into pasta sauce or offer on the side or add into risottos

Frozen Mediterranean veg medley: add to a lasagne or offer on the side with a drizzle of olive oil

Frozen forest fruits: use them in puddings, add them to yoghurt as a snack or stir into cereals and porridge

Tinned pears/peaches: make into a pudding (see page 186), offer as a snack with some yoghurt and oats, or stir into brekkie

Raisins and apricots: add to one-pot meals to add some sweetness, use in baking products

MISCELLANEOUS

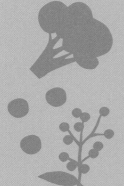

Long-life milks and milk alternatives: use for emergency milks!

Peanut butter: use in porridge, on toast, for baking instead of butter, to add fats to any dish. Mix with yoghurt for a great dip!

Marmite: save this for the toast!

Pesto: I often make my own, but an emergency jar is always useful with pasta or to stir into sauces and soups

Seasonal Ingredients Calendar

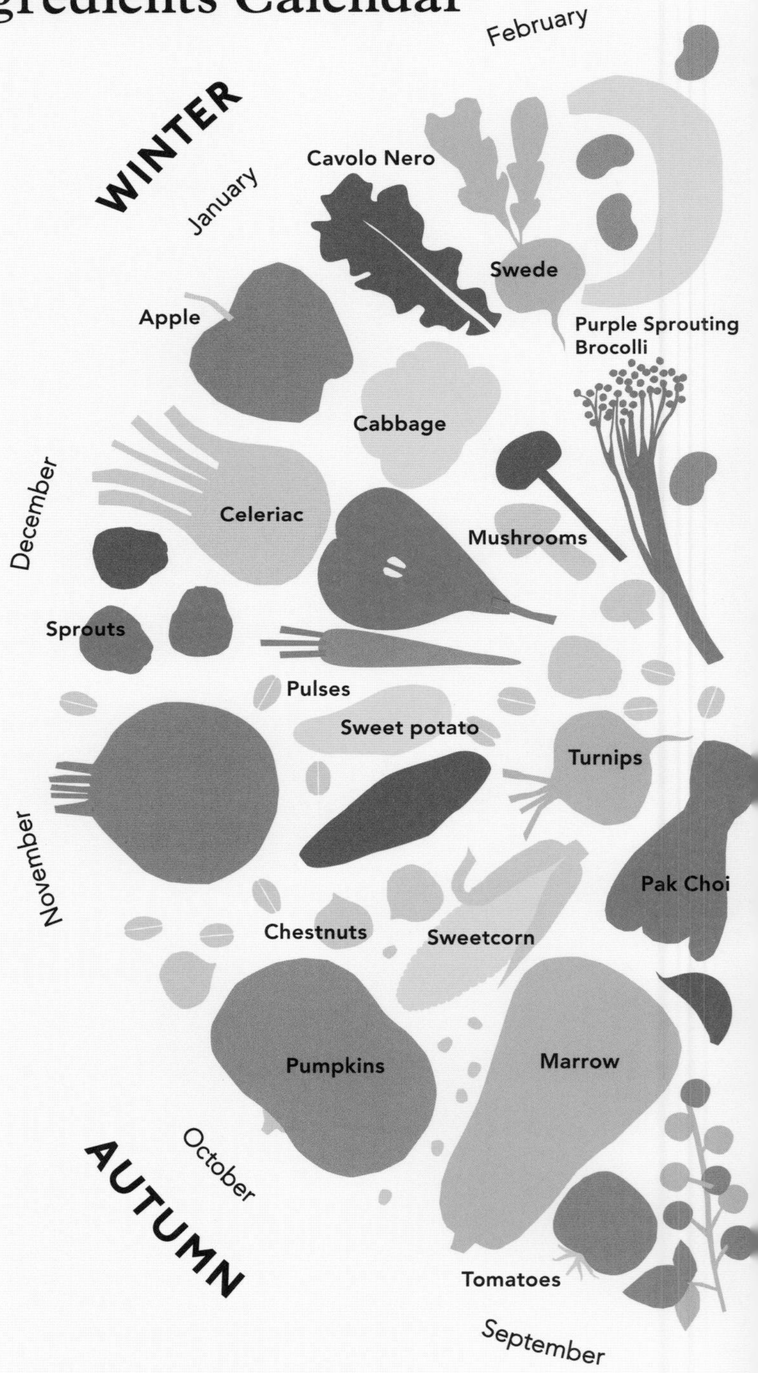

February

WINTER

January

Cavolo Nero

Swede

Purple Sprouting
Brocolli

Apple

Cabbage

December

Celeriac

Mushrooms

Sprouts

Pulses

Sweet potato

Turnips

November

Pak Choi

Chestnuts

Sweetcorn

Pumpkins

Marrow

October

AUTUMN

Tomatoes

September

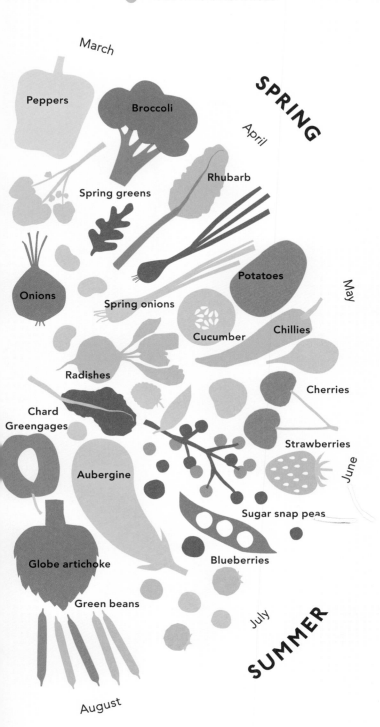

March

SPRING

Peppers

Broccoli

April

Rhubarb

Spring greens

Potatoes

May

Onions

Spring onions

Cucumber

Chillies

Radishes

Cherries

Chard
Greengages

Strawberries

June

Aubergine

Sugar snap peas

Globe artichoke

Blueberries

Green beans

July

SUMMER

August

Adding Extras to Your Family Meals

BREAKFAST

Pack it all into a smoothie

Vary your toast toppings

Make eggy bread and then add your toppings

Stir in nut butters – vary the types of these too

LUNCH

Add beans or lentils into soups and sauces

Halve the meat in recipes and swap for plant-based proteins

Add a simple side salad to any lunch

Use frozen veggies to bulk out a meal

DINNER

Serve veggies as a starter to help get plenty in

Grate veggies into soups and sauces

Add a few sprinkles of extra herbs to your dinner

Add some finger foods on the side of dinner to add extra variety

SNACKS

Combine food groups to balance snacks

Vary and avoid only offering the same few options

Use dips to add extra colour and nutrients

Make 'mini' meals like small sandwiches or leftover pasta

Use fruits (or veg like carrots) to top cereals and porridge 	Add a piece of fruit on the side	Sprinkle oats into yoghurt or on top of your cereal	Use plain yoghurt and add your own flavours 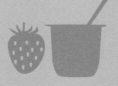
Mash avocado and add it as a dip on the side	Stir nut butters in to add flavours	Offer a choice of toppings to get kids more involved	Add mustard, tahini, lemon juice and hummus to dressings to add extra flavour and nutrients 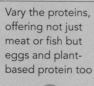
Use a few different veggies in a dish, instead of just one 	Use wholegrain versions of your fave carbs such as pasta, bread and rice 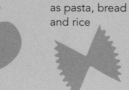	Offer a buffet spread and go to town on the colour/options available	Vary the proteins, offering not just meat or fish but eggs and plant-based protein too
Add veg sticks to whatever you're serving 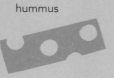	Stir through some yoghurt/ cheese or hummus	Use extras when baking, e.g. extra eggs, wholegrains or veggies.	Get kids to help you make their snacks and give them a variety to choose from 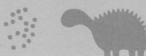

4

RECIPES

These recipes are a little different to the recipes in my other books. I've made them family friendly, so you'll see a few more ingredients that contain salt and sugar here and there – they don't appear a lot though, because I'm a real believer that we don't need huge amounts of salt and sugar to make recipes taste good.

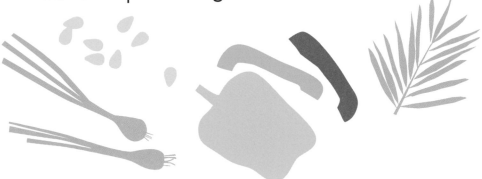

In fact, I often try foods when I'm out and about and feel that the high sugar or salt content can really overpower the flavours and stop you from tasting lots of the other delicious ingredients included in a dish.

I've indicated where you can reduce or remove the salt and sugar from recipes for younger babies and toddlers, but it's really what works for you.

The majority of the recipes in this book are simple and time and budget friendly. There are some longer ones which I've included because they are really quite special. If a meal is not plant based, they are easily adapted.

At the beginning of the Breakfast, Lunch and Dinner sections, the first **5 recipes are speedy meals,** to make your recipe search a little easier.

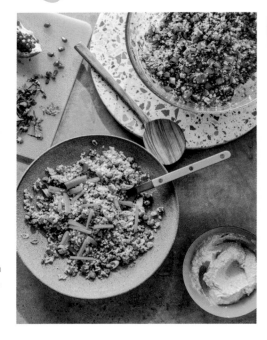

I've included a few fairly quirky dishes in this recipe section. I've loved experimenting and using ingredients that you might not expect to be put together (Monster Breakfast Baps, anyone?), or that I don't normally use in my family cooking – it's great to be experimental with recipes and I hope you enjoy doing some 'taste tests' in the kitchen as I have with my little family.

I created these recipes at a time when Ada seemed to have reached peak fussiness, so some of them were rejected by her on first go, but she's gently taken to them the more familiar they've become. Raffy has been a good recipe checker for me, as he's a lot more experimental than Ada, loves most things and isn't afraid to give new things a go. I've also tried them with my wider family and some best friends – it provided great excuses for multiple dinner parties – and they've all been such a hit! I really hope you love them too. Don't forget to refer to the Alternative Ingredients section on page 108 for simple ingredient swaps, and check out Useful Equipment on the next page to see (more or less) the kinds of equipment you'll need at home for most of the recipes in this book.

Happy Eating!

I've made the first 5 recipes in the breakfast, lunch and dinner sections '**Speedy Recipes**' so you can always easily access some of the quickest recipes.

RECIPE SYMBOLS

 Quick Prep

 Vegan

 Vegetarian

 Easily Adaptable

 No-Cook

 Ideal for Lunch Boxes

❄ Freezable

HOB

MICROWAVE

MEASURING SPOONS

CHOPPING BOARDS

MIXING BOWLS

COLANDER

KETTLE

SHARP KNIVES

OVEN

HELPFUL EQUIPMENT FOR

MIXING SPOON

FRYING PAN

WOK

FREEZER BAGS: MULTIPLE SIZES

VEGETABLE PEELER

SILICONE CUPCAKE CASES

GARLIC CRUSHER

BAKING PAPER

GRIDDLE PAN

CASSEROLE DISH

BAKING TRAY

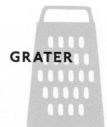

GRATER

TIN OPENER

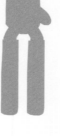

POTATO MASHER

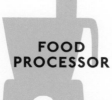

FOOD PROCESSOR

SPATULA/ FISH SLICE

KITCHEN ROLL

POTS AND PANS: VARIOUS SIZES

RECIPES IN THIS BOOK

ROLLING PIN

ELECTRIC WHISK

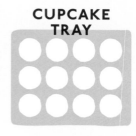

CUPCAKE TRAY

CAKE TIN

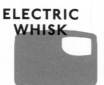

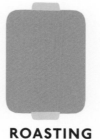

ROASTING TIN

MEASURING JUG

FREEZER- SAFE TUPPERWARE

HAND WHISK

SPOONS

Alternative Ingredients/Substitutes

INGREDIENT	ALTERNATIVE	NOTES
Eggs	Flaxseed or chia seed egg Egg replacement (from shop) 1 banana Apple sauce Tofu	1 tbsp chia seeds or ground flaxseed mixed with 3 tbsp warm water. Sit for 5 minutes until thickened. Banana/apple sauce in sweet bakery products. Instead of scrambled egg
Fresh herbs	Dried herbs	Roughly ⅓–¼ of the amount needed
Milk	Usually any plant-based alternatives work well.	Some are more-watery, so may not thicken products as well. Aim for plain and fortified.
Fish	Swap for tofu, butter beans, chickpeas or chicken. Add avocado, olive oil for some omega-3 fatty acids.	These alternatives won't work in all recipes, and often don't have the same flavour/texture, but can replace some of the nutrients.
Cheese	Nutritional yeast Dairy-free cheese Tofu	These don't replace the texture, but can add a cheesy flavour. Dairy-free cheese can work well, but it takes a bit of trial and error to find a good one.
Meat	Tofu Lentils Beans Chickpeas Quorn	Tofu if in chunks Lots of these can replace the nutrients in meat, but not the texture/flavours. It's always good to vary the plant-based protein/iron sources you use in foods.
Tofu	Meat Chicken Fish Quorn Beans Eggs	If you're not a tofu fan, simply swap it out in the recipe for any of these. Meat, chicken and fish will need to be cooked to packet instructions.
Quinoa	Couscous Buckwheat Rice Potatoes	Grains are super easy to swap so don't be afraid to swap it and follow packet instructions to ensure it's cooked.

INGREDIENT	ALTERNATIVE	NOTES
Milled seeds	N/A	There aren't really any suitable substitutes for milled seeds, but quite often you can simply leave them out or add a little more dry matter e.g., flour to compensate.
Pasta	Any other style of pasta Rice or couscous Gnocchi Spiralised veg	These can all work well as replacements, but remember that spiralised veggies aren't a replacement for carbs, nutritionally, but they can be a great, fresh alternative sometimes
Plain flour	Gluten-free flour Ground almonds Polenta	Easy to swap these like for like in many recipes.
Self-raising flour	Plain flour and baking powder	Add 2 teaspoons of baking powder to 150g plain flour
Butter	Plant-based spreads Olive oil	Plant-based spreads and olive oil usually work just as well as butter in cooking. Vary the types of fats you use.
Soured cream	Yoghurt Crème fraîche	These usually work well as substitutes.
Beans	Different types of beans and chickpeas can be pretty much interchangeable. You can also swap beans for tofu or small chunks of chicken or fish.	Mixed beans can be a good way to add even more of a variety.
Garlic powder	Garlic flakes Garlic clove	The equivalent for ½ teaspoon of garlic powder is 1 fresh garlic clove
Root veggies	Carrot/parsnips/butternut squash can be used interchangeably. Use frozen vegetable varieties as well.	Some harder veg takes longer to cook, so you might need to take this into account in the cooking time. Add frozen veggies in at the end of the recipe.
Peanut butters	Any other nut butter Tahini No-Nuts nut butter (you can find online) Seed butters e.g., sunflower butter Dairy butter or spread	

Breakfast

EASY FAMILY SMOOTHIE

As my children have grown older, I've found that smoothies make a great quick breakfast. We usually have them alongside something else, as a filling start to the day. I like to make smoothies a really balanced option, so you aren't just having a dose of fruit and nothing more. We're always adding greens, proteins and some dairy or dairy-free alternatives into ours. This smoothie recipe is a weekend staple in our house and Ada is a huge fan!

Serves: 4 (makes about 600ml)
Prep time: 5 minutes

45g porridge oats
250ml milk of choice
generous handful of spinach,
    washed (about 30g)
1 tbsp nut butter (e.g., almond)
1 ripe banana, peeled
150g mixed frozen fruit (such
    as berries and/or mango)

1. Pop the oats, then the milk, and the rest of the ingredients, into a blender and blitz until smooth. Add a little more milk if you prefer.

2. Divide between glasses or cups and serve.

APPLE CRUMBLE BIRCHER

In my house we are big porridge fans. This no-cook recipe is a super quick breakfast option that is a delicious and speedy alternative to porridge. And it's ready in seconds! You can easily double it up to make a big batch, so you have plenty for the week. It's sweet, creamy and easy to adapt, so that's a winner in my book!

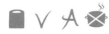

Makes: about 600g of bircher (enough for a family of 4, with leftovers)
Prep time: 10 minutes, plus overnight soaking

100g porridge oats
100g natural yoghurt or
    dairy-free yoghurt alternative
350ml milk of choice
1 apple, peeled and grated
¼ tsp ground cinnamon
¼ tsp ground ginger
¼ tsp ground nutmeg
1 tsp vanilla extract (optional)

TO SERVE (OPTIONAL)
finely chopped nuts (hazelnuts
    and almonds are good)
fresh berries
1 apple, thinly sliced
yoghurt of choice

1. The night before, mix all the ingredients together in an airtight container, then chill.
2. The next morning, give the bircher a stir and spoon into bowls, then top with some finely chopped nuts, fresh berries and sliced apple, and an extra dollop of yoghurt if you want to.

For babies and young children:
Avoid whole and chopped nuts until toddlers have developed full eating skills, so ideally grind and add these on for younger children or just leave this topping off.

Make ahead: The bircher will keep in the fridge, sealed in an airtight container, for up to 2–3 days.

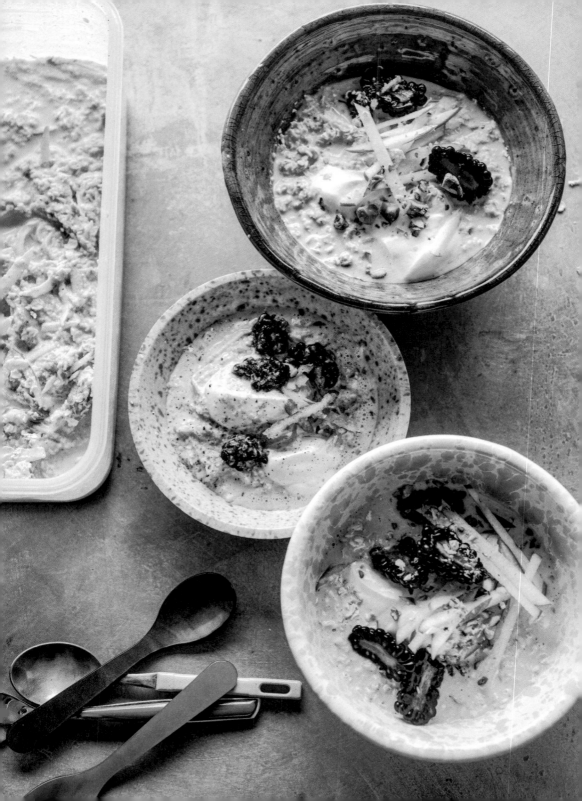

SPEEDY

BLUEBERRY BREAKFAST MUFFINS

I'm a huge fan of blueberry muffins, and this is a healthy, family friendly version. These juicy muffins are perfect for breakfast or on-the-go snacks. The basic recipe isn't very sweet, so if you're looking for an extra sweet kick add a couple of teaspoons of sugar to the mix. My two like these without the added sugar, especially served with some yoghurt on the side. They also freeze brilliantly, so you can batch-bake and defrost them individually the night before you want to eat them. Spelt flour adds extra nutrients and a nutty flavour, but it's completely optional.

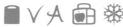

Makes: 12 muffins
Prep time: 5–10 minutes
Cook time: 25–30 minutes

120g self-raising flour
50g plain wholemeal flour or spelt flour
50g milled seeds: e.g. chia, flax, pumpkin
1 tsp baking powder
2 tsp sugar (optional)
180ml fresh apple juice (not from concentrate)
2 medium free-range eggs (or
    2 chia seed eggs – see page 108)
1 ripe banana, peeled and mashed
1 tsp vanilla extract
50ml mild olive or sunflower oil,
    or melted butter
200g fresh or frozen blueberries
3 tbsp maple syrup or agave
    syrup, for brushing (optional)

1. Preheat the oven to 200°C/180°C fan, and line a 12-hole muffin tin with paper or silicone cases.
2. Put the flours, seeds and baking powder (and sugar, if using) into a medium mixing bowl, and put the apple juice, eggs, banana, vanilla extract and oil or melted butter into a measuring jug.
3. Whisk the wet ingredients together until well combined, then pour into the flour bowl and add the blueberries. Mix everything together until just combined (don't overmix or the muffins will be tough), then divide evenly among the 12 cases – you can fill them quite full.
4. Bake in the oven for 25–30 minutes until golden and risen. If you're using the syrup, brush the tops of the muffins as soon as they come out of the oven.
5. Leave to cool in the tin for 5–10 minutes (this allows them to firm up a little), then carefully remove to a cooling rack and leave to cool completely or until just warm.
6. They're best eaten on the day they're baked, but they'll keep in a tin somewhere cool and dry for up to 3 days.

For babies and young children:
Leave out the sugar and syrup – the blueberries add plenty of sweetness and some juiciness. These are great for babies who are experimenting with finger foods – simply slice them into long shapes and allow baby to self-feed.

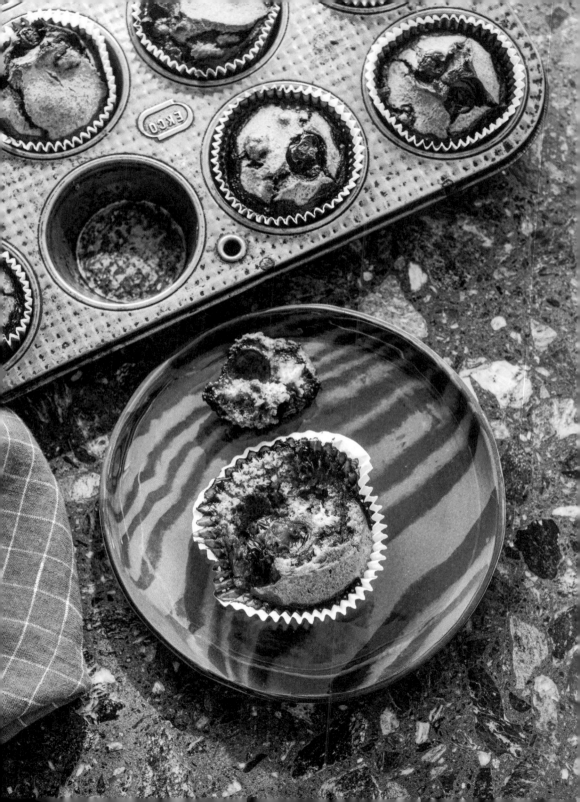

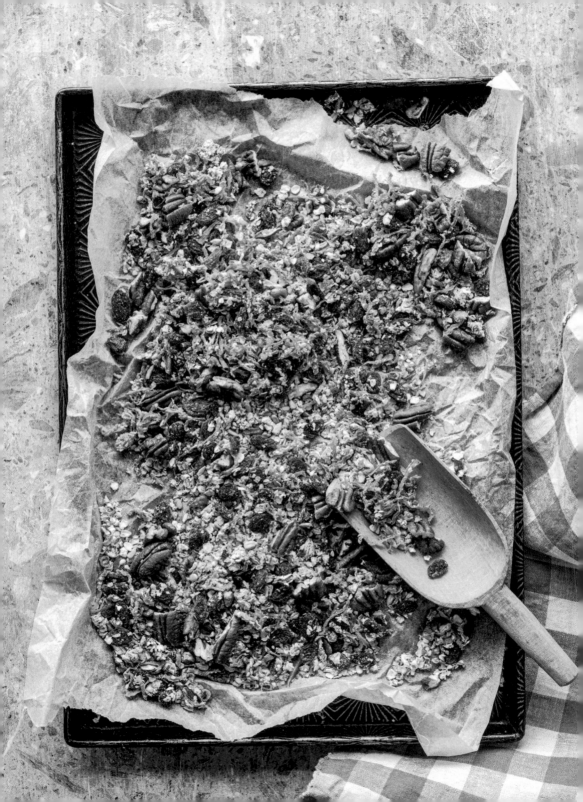

CARROT CAKE GRANOLA

I have a granola recipe in *How to Feed Your Toddler*, but wanted to experiment with a carrot version, and I think this might be one of my favourite recipes! All the flavours of a carrot cake, in a no-added-sugar granola that is such a hit and really doesn't need the added sugar that you get in shop-bought granola. This has fast become a go-to breakfast recipe in my house.

Makes: enough to fill a 1-litre jar
Prep time: 5 minutes
Cook time: 35 minutes

150g porridge oats
250g carrots, peeled and
    coarsely grated
100g pecans, roughly
    chopped or ground
½ tsp ground cinnamon
¼ tsp ground nutmeg
finely grated zest and juice
    of 1 orange
50g mixed seeds or 30g
    milled seeds
120g sultanas

1. Preheat the oven to 170°C/150°C fan and line two large baking trays with non-stick baking paper. Mix all the ingredients together in a large mixing bowl, then massage everything with your hands so the orange juice evenly coats everything.
2. Spread the mixture out over the lined baking trays, then bake for 15 minutes.
3. Turn the oven down to 150°C/130°C fan and stir the granola to move the bits from the edges to the middle and vice versa. Spread it all back out again, then return to the oven and bake for another 20 minutes, or until the oats are completely crisp and the kitchen smells of orange and spice.
4. Remove from the oven, leave to cool completely on the tray, then transfer to a 1-litre storage container and keep somewhere cool and dry. The granola will keep for up to 2 weeks.

**For babies
and young children:**
This one might not be ideal for babies as it has some harder textures.

For little ones, grind up the pecans, and swap the mixed seeds for 30g milled seeds, so that there are no chunks in the mixture. You could chop the sultanas for small children too.

SPEEDY

EASY TOAST
TOPPERS

Each makes: 1 slice
of topped toast
Prep time: 5 minutes

I love toast for a simple breakfast, but sometimes I like to think outside the box with what I serve on top. I'm always talking about adding extras in recipes, so here is an example of how you can do this simply. These are more for inspo than anything, but my two are loving the banana, blueberry and nut butter one, it's fast become a breakfast staple! These are great alternatives to toast and jam, and can all be whipped up in 5 minutes flat.

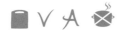

SUNSHINE SCRAMBLED EGGS

1. Whisk 1 medium free-range egg with a pinch each of turmeric and ground cumin using a fork. Melt a knob of unsalted butter or a drizzle of olive oil in a small non-stick frying pan over a medium-high heat, and when the butter sizzles (or the oil shimmers), add the egg.
2. Stir slowly with a spatula to scramble the eggs until they're almost set, then set aside – they'll finish cooking in the residual heat. Butter a slice of wholemeal toast, then top with the eggs. Adults and older children might like a few sprigs of coriander and a squeeze of lemon juice to serve.

SMASHED AVOCADO AND CHIVE

1. Scoop half a ripe avocado into a small bowl with a squeeze of lime juice and 5 finely chopped chives. Mash roughly with a fork, then spread on a slice of wholemeal toast (buttered if you like), and top with 3 more roughly snipped chives.
2. Serve immediately, adding a sprinkle of dried chilli flakes for adults, if you like.

BANANA, BLUEBERRY
AND NUTTY BUTTER

1. Slice half a banana and 5 blueberries. Spread a slice of wholemeal toast with 2 teaspoons of nut butter (we like peanut) then arrange the banana and blueberry slices over the top.
2. If serving adults or older children, a drizzle of maple syrup or honey is also delicious. Squash the blueberries a little for babies and young children.

CARROT AND POTATO ROSTIS

These are a little fiddly, but super delicious. They are pretty simple but can be fragile on the pan. Try to get them nice and crispy before you flip them, and this can really help them stay together. They're best made with old potatoes, so it's great for spuds that need using up. I love the flavour combinations of the toppings on these, they work perfectly. You can always roast the tomatoes if you have the time.

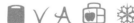

Makes: 10 rostis (3 each for adults/teens, 2 each for little ones)
Prep time: 10 minutes
Cook time: 20–30 minutes

150g carrots, peeled and grated
350g floury potatoes (older is best), peeled
2 tbsp mild or light olive oil or 30g unsalted melted butter, plus extra oil for frying

TO SERVE
2 ripe avocados, destoned and sliced
12 cherry tomatoes, quartered
1 sprig of mint, leaves picked and thinly sliced
sprinkle of feta cheese (optional)
lime wedges

1. Put the carrots in a sieve, then pop into a large mixing bowl.
2. Grate the potatoes into the bowl of carrot then put the mixture in a clean tea towel, wrap it and give it a tight squeeze to remove excess liquid.
3. Put the mixture back in the bowl, add the olive oil or melted butter and toss together with your hands. Add a pinch of salt if you like – it will draw the starch out of the potatoes and help the rostis stick together. Put a large, non-stick frying pan over a medium heat and drizzle in a little oil.
4. Once the veg are well combined, turn the heat up to medium-high. Take a small handful of the mixture and gently place it into the pan, pressing into a thin disc that's roughly 10cm diameter. Repeat with more handfuls of the mixture (you'll probably need to fry them in batches).
5. Cook for about 10 minutes, pressing the tops down gently to flatten, until the underside is deep golden and crisp – you might need to add a little extra oil. When you see the edges brown, carefully flip the rostis with a fish slice, turn the heat down to medium-low and cook for another 10 minutes, pressing them down from time to time to release the moisture. Once cooked, drain on kitchen paper and keep warm on a lined baking tray while you cook the rest.
6. Plate up 2–3 rostis per serving with some sliced avocado and cherry tomatoes, and a scatter of sliced mint and feta, if using. Serve with lime wedges for squeezing.

BAKED BANANA BARS

I love an on-the-go breakfast idea and these porridge bars have been such a hit with my kids. They work well as a snack too, and are very easy to put together. They take a little time on the cooking front, but next to no time to prep, and are well worth it. They freeze well so are perfect for batch-cooking.

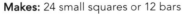

Makes: 24 small squares or 12 bars
Prep time: 5 minutes
Cook time: 50–55 minutes

100g porridge oats
180ml milk of choice
2 large, very ripe bananas (around 200g in total)
85g sultanas (or raisins, chopped dates, chopped dried apricots)
½ tsp mixed spice (or ground cinnamon or nutmeg)
3 tbsp mixed seeds (ground for babies/toddlers)

1. Preheat the oven to 180°C/160°C fan and line a 20cm square shallow baking tin with non-stick baking paper. Mix all the ingredients together (except the seeds), then mash it well with a fork to completely break up the bananas. Once everything is well mixed, scoop it into the baking tin and level the top. Sprinkle the mixed seeds on top (leave off or grind if serving to babies and young children).
2. Bake for 50–55 minutes, until the top is golden and crisp. Once cooked, remove from the tin using the baking paper and leave to cool on a rack until either warm or cooled to room temperature.
3. Slice into 24 small squares, or 12 larger bars to serve. The bars will keep in an airtight container for up to 3 days, or can be wrapped in cling film/beeswax and frozen individually, then defrosted on the counter overnight ready for the morning. You can also reheat them uncovered in a microwave for 30 seconds if you'd like them warm.

For babies and young children: They should be okay with the texture of these as soon as they have moved on to slightly more complex finger foods. Avoid whole seeds, offer them ground instead, or simply leave them off any of the bars/squares that are for your baby/toddler.

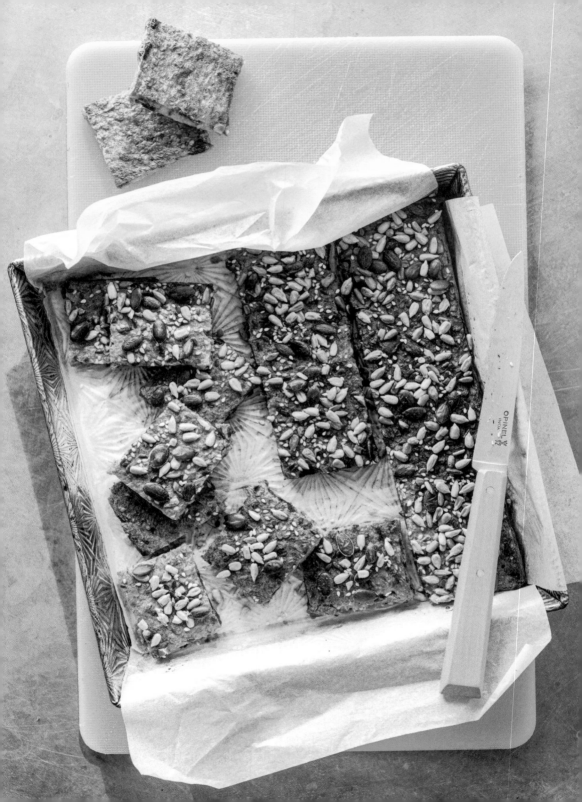

FLUFFY COCONUT PANCAKES

This is an easy, egg-free pancake recipe. Everyone loves a pancake in my house, and we often have them at the weekend. This American-style recipe produces super-fluffy pancakes with a mild coconutty flavour, and they are easy to freeze for later.

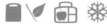

Makes: 10–12 pancakes
Prep time: 10 minutes
Cook time: 15 minutes

120g self-raising flour (wholemeal if possible)
30g porridge oats
40g desiccated coconut, plus a little extra to serve
220g milk of choice (try light coconut milk if you want extra coconutty flavour)
1 flaxseed egg (see page 108) or 1 large free-range egg
2 tbsp olive oil

TO SERVE
120g frozen fruits (or any fruits you have that need using up)
160g coconut yoghurt (or any yoghurt will do)
maple syrup (optional)

1. Mix the flour, porridge oats and desiccated coconut in a bowl then gradually stir in the milk and the thickened flaxseed egg/egg, mixing until smooth.
2. Put a large frying pan over a medium heat, add a little of the oil then add 5–6 individual heaped tablespoons of pancake batter to the pan (depending the size of your pan, you might need to cook the pancakes in 2–3 batches) and cook for 2–3 minutes on each side, or until golden and cooked through. Set to one side and cook the remaining batter.
3. Pop the frozen fruit into the microwave in a microwave-safe bowl for 2–3 minutes to make a super-quick fruit topping.
4. Serve a couple of pancakes per person with a dollop of yoghurt, a drizzle of fruit and a drizzle of maple syrup and extra desiccated coconut if that appeals!

For babies and young children: Leave out the maple syrup.

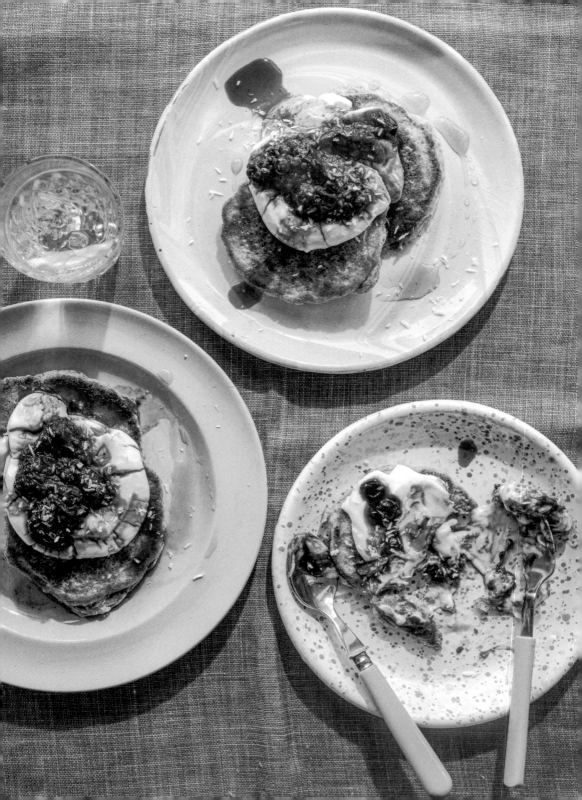

ORANGEY BREAKFAST WAFFLES

These easy waffles make a great alternative to pancakes, but you don't need a waffle maker. They were an instant hit when testing them at home. Top them with whatever fruit you like, but they work so well with chopped/ground pecans and orange slices. For adults and older kids, a little maple syrup will work well too!

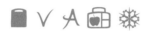

Makes: 2 large waffles, serves 4
Prep time: 10–20 minutes
Cook time: 15–20 minutes

150g self-raising flour
finely grated zest of 2 clementines or
   1 orange (keep the whole fruit to serve)
1 medium free-range egg or chia seed egg
   (see page 108)
240ml milk of choice
60g unsalted butter or dairy-free
   alternative, melted

TO SERVE
the whole clementines or orange
   from zesting above
25g pecans or other nuts, finely chopped
   or ground
yoghurt of choice (I used Greek)
maple syrup/honey for adults and older
   kids (optional)

Cook's tip: If you want to create a square pattern on your waffles, carefully turn them 90-degrees halfway through their first cooking time and cook for 2–3 minutes more before flipping them. Try not to move them once they're turned, so the bar marks stay sharp.

1. Put a non-stick griddle pan over a medium-high heat while you make the batter. Put the flour and citrus zest into a medium mixing bowl and stir together. Beat the egg (or chia seed egg), milk and melted butter together in a separate bowl or jug until the mixture is smooth, then gradually pour it into the flour, whisking with a fork as you go, until you have a thick, smooth liquid. Depending on the size of your egg, you might need to add a little more milk – the mixture should be just a bit thicker than double cream.

2. Once the griddle pan is hot, splash a drop of cooking oil into the pan and pour half the batter in. If necessary, smooth it down with a fork, until it covers most of the surface (it should be about 5mm thick). Turn the heat down to medium and cook for 3–4 minutes, until the underside is deep golden and crisp, and the top has bubbled then solidified and lost its sheen.

3. Carefully flip the waffle over and cook for another 3–4 minutes, turning the heat down to low if the waffle is colouring too much. Once cooked, slide the waffle onto a plate and make the second waffle with the rest of the batter.

4. To serve, peel the zested clementines or orange and slice into thin rounds, adding some extra fruit in if you'd like more. Cut the waffles into quarters, then add a dollop of yoghurt, some fruit slices, a scattering of chopped nuts (leave off or grind for babies/toddlers) and a squeeze of clementine to finish.

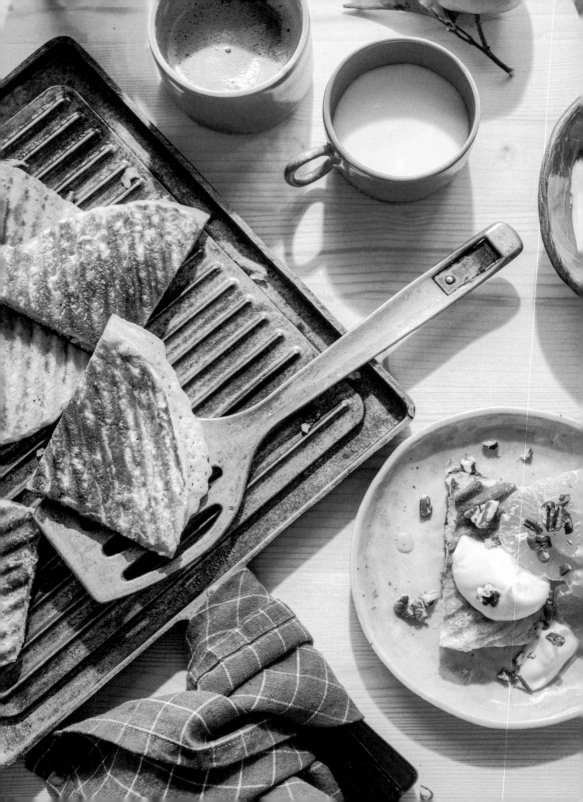

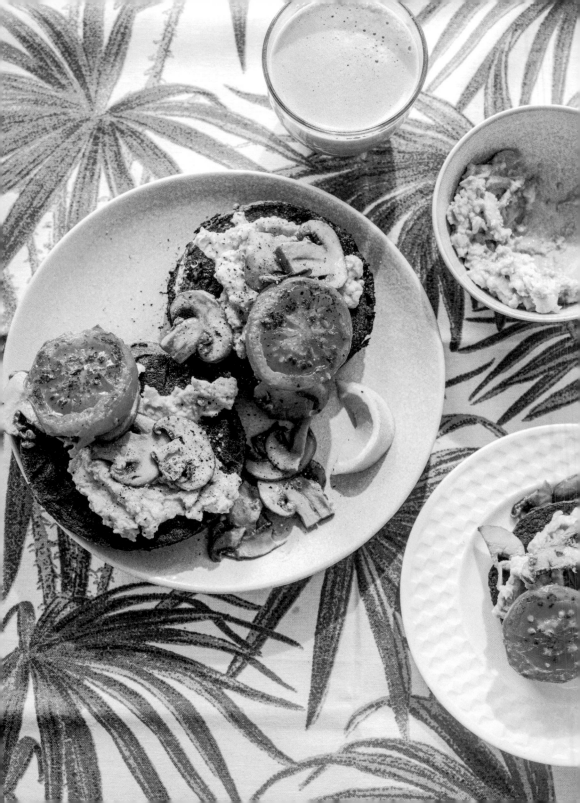

MONSTER BREAKFAST BAPS

I love this recipe. It's totally whacky but really delicious, and a completely different breakfast to any I've created before. The green muffins are such a novelty – hopefully your family will love them too! You can always change up the veggies that go on top, or leave them out completely. If you want to leave out the egg it still works, but it won't go as crispy when fried without it.

Serves: 4
Prep time: 15 minutes
Cook time: 10–15 minutes

40g unsalted butter, plus extra for spreading
1 garlic clove, peeled and crushed/chopped
200g spinach, washed
4 English muffins, halved
4 medium ripe tomatoes, halved
handful of chestnut mushrooms, thinly sliced
splash of milk of choice
2 large free-range eggs
1 ripe avocado, mashed (optional)
½ lemon (optional)

For babies and young children: Let them dissect the baps or cut them into thin strips for them to help themselves.

1. Melt half the butter in a large frying pan over a medium heat, add the garlic and cook for a few minutes, then add the spinach and cook, stirring, for 5 minutes until wilted. Pop the halved muffins in the toaster to get them a little golden.
2. Transfer the spinach and garlic to a blender. Keep the pan on the hob and add the remaining butter, then add the halved tomatoes and mushrooms and cook gently over a medium heat for 5 minutes until golden, stirring occasionally.
3. To make the green egg mix, add the milk to the blender and whizz until the mixture is green and thick, then crack in the eggs and mix again briefly to combine. Pour this mix into a shallow bowl.
4. Dunk the toasted muffins into the green egg mix on both sides to coat them completely. Hold them up and shake off any excess. Remove the mushrooms and tomatoes from the frying pan and set aside, then add the coated muffins to the frying pan with a little oil and cook for 3–4 minutes on each side until browning a little.
5. Plate up. Mix the mashed avocado with a little squeeze of lemon then dollop onto the muffins, then add the cooked mushrooms and tomatoes. Serve straight away.

Lunch

QUICK VEGGIE FRITTATA

Everyone needs a quick go-to recipe for an emergency meal and this works so well. It takes 20 minutes from beginning to end, and is so versatile. It can be cooled, cut up for lunchboxes, and can be made with whatever your favourite frozen veg mix is (you can make it dairy-free, too).

 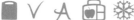

Serves: 3–4
Prep and cook time: 20 minutes

25g unsalted butter or 1½ tbsp olive oil
125g quick-cook frozen vegetables
    (I used a pea and bean medley)
6 large free-range eggs, beaten well
30g mature cheddar cheese, grated,
    or 2 tbsp nutritional yeast flakes

1. Heat the grill to high, and put the butter or oil into a non-stick 20cm (across the top) frying pan along with the frozen vegetables, and place over a medium heat. Allow the butter to melt or the oil to heat and the vegetables to start to sizzle, then cook, stirring often, for 3–4 minutes, until the vegetables have completely defrosted.
2. Spread them out evenly around the pan, then mix the cheese or yeast with the eggs and gently pour the mixture into the pan. Cook for 5–6 minutes, until the sides have set and are shrinking away from the pan, but the middle of the mixture is still liquid.
3. Transfer to the hot grill and cook for another 2–3 minutes, keeping an eye on it, until the top is set and you can't see any liquid when you tilt the pan. Once cooked, carefully invert it onto a serving board, then cut up into wedges to serve.

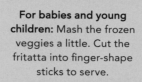

For babies and young children: Mash the frozen veggies a little. Cut the fritatta into finger-shape sticks to serve.

Make ahead: Make the frittata, cool and keep chilled in an airtight container for up to 2 days.

SPEEDY

CORONATION TOFU WRAP

I've made this take on the classic Coronation chicken recipe vegan, but you can swap the tofu for cooked, shredded chicken (it's a perfect way to use up Sunday roast leftovers), and swap the yoghurt for regular Greek. The flavours really go together so well. It's a great way to offer tofu to the family with plenty of other flavours added in. If you have more time you can always roast the drained tofu a little in the oven to crisp and heat it up.

Makes: enough for about 4 wraps
Prep time: 10 minutes

300g firm tofu, cut into bite-sized chunks
150g coconut yoghurt (or use your
    favourite dairy-free yoghurt)
6 sprigs of coriander, finely chopped
1½–2 tsp mild or medium curry powder,
    to taste
large pinch of turmeric
big squeeze of lemon juice
4 tbsp fresh pomegranate seeds
    (or use finely chopped mango
    or raisins/sultanas)

TO SERVE
4 tortilla wraps, warmed through
little gem lettuce, shredded

1. Put the tofu chunks on 2–3 layers of kitchen paper. Press down gently to drain off some of the excess liquid.
2. Meanwhile, mix the yoghurt, coriander, curry powder, turmeric and lemon juice together in a medium mixing bowl.
3. Once the tofu has drained, gently stir it through the yoghurt mix, adding the pomegranate seeds (or other fruit), then pile into warmed wraps with some little gem lettuce. Season the adults' versions if you like (I think it's fine without!), then roll up and eat immediately.

For babies and young children: This recipe is nice and soft, but young babies might struggle with the wrap and lettuce – you could offer it in pitta sticks instead, or cut the filled wrap into rounds, which might be easier for babies to manage. Also, the pomegranate seeds might be too much for babies as they are tough to crunch.

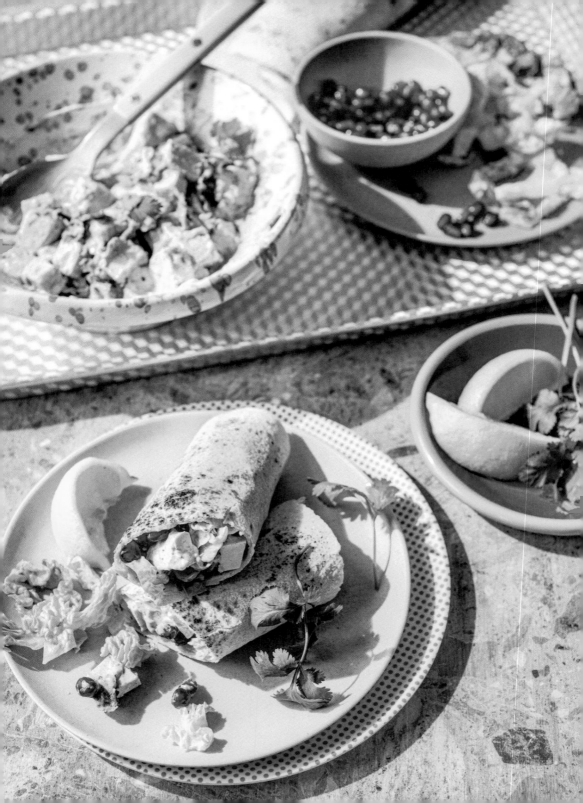

SALMON PATÉ ON TOAST

I always love having a store-cupboard staple option for when I'm out of ideas for lunch at home with the kids. This is such a simple lunch to whip up and is quick, and no-cook. You can easily use dairy-free alternatives to cream cheese, and I sometimes make it with other types of fish, depending on what tins I have in the cupboard.

Makes: about 270g – enough for 4 people for lunch with a little left over
Prep time: 5 minutes

213g tin wild salmon, skinless and
    boneless, oil drained
60g cream cheese
finely grated zest of ½ lemon, plus juice
    to taste and extra zest to garnish
3 sprigs of dill, stalks removed (or ¼ tsp
    of dried dill), plus a few extra for garnish

TO SERVE
wholemeal or seeded toast,
    buttered if you like
watercress sprigs (optional)
sliced cucumber (optional)
lemon wedges (optional)
black pepper (optional)

1. Put the salmon, cream cheese, half the lemon's zest and a big squeeze of lemon juice into a food processor (or use a hand blender/potato masher), whiz to combine. Taste, and add the dill and some extra lemon juice if you would like it sharper. Blitz again until almost smooth.

2. Spread a layer of salmon over toast, then slice into fingers.

3. Serve immediately, with watercress and/or cucumber, some extra lemon zest grated on top, a few dill sprigs and a twist of black pepper.

For babies and young children:
This is a great one for babies, leave off some of the extra toppings like the pepper, watercress and dill, and go a little easy on the sharp lemon. Cut into finger sticks for self-feeding.

SWEET AND SAVOURY GRAINS

This works well as a light and easy lunch option, and you can easily combine it with proteins such as chickpeas, fish or boiled eggs. It also works so well as a side or base for other recipes. The sweet version goes particularly well with the tagine on page 173.

Makes: 2 large bowls
Prep time: 5–10 minutes plus grain cooking time
Cook time: Variable, grain dependent
Start with 150g couscous, rice or bulgur wheat and cook to packet instructions.

FOR THE SWEET DISH
Stir through the cooked grains:

20g fresh soft herbs (parsley, coriander or mint, or a combination), leaves picked and finely chopped
1 red pepper, deseeded and finely diced
½ cucumber, deseeded and finely diced
100g pomegranate seeds (from about 1 whole pomegranate fruit) (optional)
2 tbsp extra-virgin olive oil
dairy-free natural yoghurt, to serve (optional)

FOR THE SAVOURY DISH
Stir through the cooked grains:

150g cooked frozen veggies e.g., peas, carrots and peppers
100g chopped roasted red peppers (can also just use a fresh chopped pepper but it doesn't add as much flavour)
1 tsp cumin seeds
big dollop of natural yoghurt or hummus, to serve (optional)

For babies and young children:
Leave out the pomegranate seeds and chop the veggies very small. Give their portions a mash with the back of a fork, if needed.

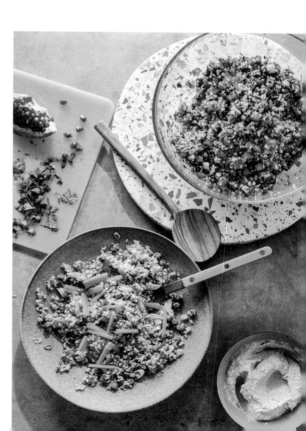

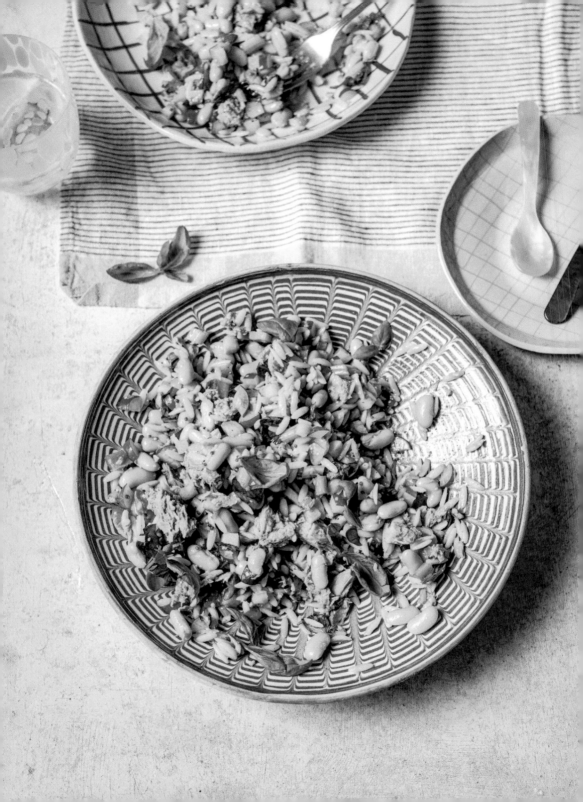

TUNA ORZO SALAD

I love this orzo salad – it's definitely one that the whole family will enjoy, and it's easy to adapt. The beans are a source of protein, so you can always leave out the tuna if you don't eat fish, or swap the orzo for another pasta, or rice. This is a lovely, summery recipe that's great for getting kids into salad – the small pieces of veg are easy to fork up and add a great crunch. Chop the vegetables as large or small as you like (smaller for little ones), but make sure all the pieces are roughly the same size.

Serves: 4
Prep time: 10–15 minutes
Cook time: 10–12 minutes (for the orzo)

125g orzo
2 celery sticks, finely diced
8 radishes, finely diced
½ cucumber, finely diced
400g tin cannellini beans, drained and rinsed
2 x 160g tins tuna in spring water
    or olive oil, drained
10g basil, leaves picked and thinly sliced,
    plus extra leaves, to garnish

FOR THE DRESSING

1 tbsp balsamic vinegar (plus extra,
    optional, for adults)
1 tbsp grainy mustard
3 tbsp mild or blended olive oil

1. Cook the orzo according to the packet instructions, then drain well. Allow to steam in the sieve for a few minutes, breaking it up with a fork so it doesn't stick together.
2. To make the dressing, put the vinegar and mustard in a small jar or bowl and whisk with a fork. Once combined and smooth, gradually whisk in the olive oil until you have a smooth, glossy dressing.
3. Mix the celery, radishes, cucumber, beans and tuna together in a bowl. Stir through the cooked orzo, then the dressing and the basil. Divide among bowls and garnish with whole basil leaves. Serve immediately, adding a little more balsamic vinegar if you like.

Make ahead: You can make the salad up to 2 days ahead and keep in the fridge. Don't dress it until about 15 minutes before serving though, or the orzo might taste a little bitter.

For babies and young children: The raw veggies might be a little tough for young babies to crunch through, depending on their eating skills. If serving for babies you can set aside some of the orzo and cucumber and mash up beans with tinned tuna for their meal.

Most children should be able to cope with these textures but younger children (1–2 years), depending on their eating skills, might need the veggies chopping very small or almost grating into the dish, and mash the beans a little too. If your little ones haven't tried vinegar or mustard before you can leave it off or just offer a small amount.

TOFU AND WATERMELON NOODLES

This recipe uses some quirky ingredients, so it's a good one for experimenting with new foods for your family. It's quick to put together and adaptable too: it works well with strips of cooked chicken instead of tofu, and it's super easy to swap ingredients in and out. I've used wholewheat noodles, but for speed you could use rice noodles that only need soaking!

Serves: 4
Prep and cook time: 15 minutes, plus draining and soaking

250g firm tofu, cut into small chunks
3 nests of medium wholewheat noodles (200g)
400g watermelon flesh, chopped into small chunks
4–5 sprigs of mint, leaves picked and finely chopped
40g roasted unsalted peanuts, chopped (or ground)
a few squirts of maple syrup (optional)
soy sauce, to taste (optional)

FOR THE DRESSING
4 tbsp sesame oil
juice of 1 lime
4 tbsp peanut butter

1. Put the tofu chunks on top of 2–3 layers of kitchen paper, and press down gently on top of them to remove any excess liquid.
2. Cook the noodles as per packet instructions then drain them and rinse under cold water.
3. To make the dressing, mix all the ingredients together.
4. Toss the drained tofu with the noodles, watermelon and most of the mint. Drizzle the dressing over and toss that through well, then garnish with the remaining mint and serve, drizzled with a little soy sauce/maple syrup (if you like) and with the peanuts mixed into the adult dishes.

This might be a very experimental one for the kids, so don't worry if they dissect it and just eat the bits they like.

For babies and young children:
Chop the noodles really well to make them more manageable, or give them a little mash with a fork. Don't offer the nuts to babies or young toddlers or grind them up before adding them to the dish. Leave out the maple syrup and soy sauce.

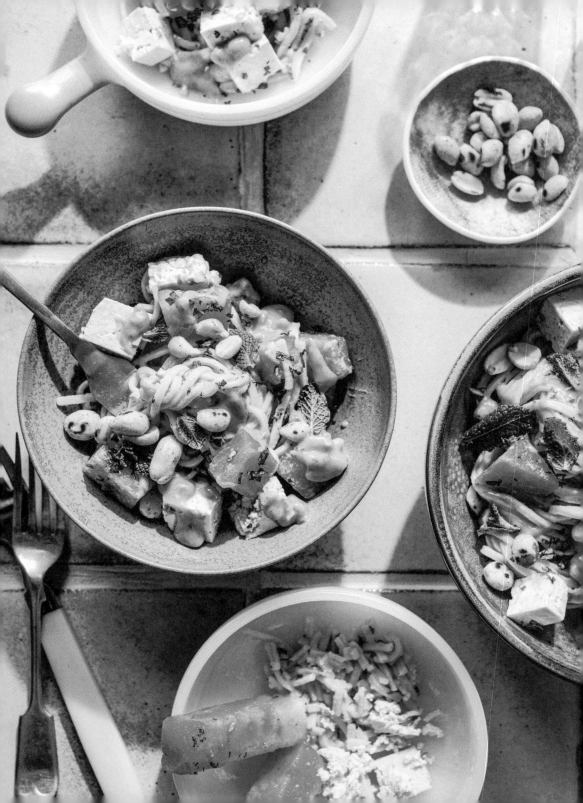

A COMFORTING CHICKEN SOUP

This is wonderful for when the family are laid low with colds or other illnesses – it's so comforting and nourishing. It takes a little longer than some of the other meals, but it makes a huge batch so it's perfect for freezing, ready for when you need some proper food TLC.

Makes: about 2.5 litres
Prep time: 20 minutes, plus cooling
Cook time: 2 hours 45 minutes

FOR THE STOCK

1.5kg whole free-range (RSPCA-approved) chicken, untrussed
2 celery sticks, broken into thirds
2 carrots, washed and roughly chopped
1 onion, quartered, skin-on
2 bay leaves

FOR THE SOUP

olive or sunflower oil, for frying
2 leeks, halved lengthways, washed and thinly sliced
2 carrots, peeled and finely diced
2 celery sticks, finely diced
150g pearl barley, well rinsed
lemon juice, to taste
finely chopped parsley, to garnish (optional)
seasoning, to taste (for adults)

> **For babies and young children:** You can easily blend into a smooth texture for younger children if needed, and leave off any added salt.

1. Preheat the oven to 160°C/140°C fan. Put the chicken breast-side down with the vegetables, bay leaves and peppercorns in a large, ovenproof, lidded pan. Pour in 3 litres of water, cover with the lid and put in the oven for 2 hours. After this time, remove the pan and leave for 1–2 hours to cool.

2. Add a drizzle of oil to a large saucepan or stock pot, place over a medium heat and fry the soup vegetables for 10 minutes, stirring often, until they are softened and a little coloured.

3. Strain the chicken stock into the pan through a sieve and add the pearl barley. Bring everything to a gentle simmer, then cook for 30 minutes, or until the barley has swollen and is tender.

4. Meanwhile, once the chicken has cooled, remove the skin and strip the meat. Discard the carcass, and tear the meat into strips. You can always set aside some of the meat to use for other meals during the week, if you don't want to use it all in this soup. As the chicken is poached the thigh meat will be very juicy – don't worry, it is cooked, it just looks different to the meat from a roast bird.

5. Stir the chicken through the soup and cook for another 5 minutes until the meat is piping hot. Remove any portions for small children, and season the rest with salt and lemon juice, if you like.

6. Ladle the soup into bowls and scatter over a little parsley. Serve immediately, or leave to cool and portion into storage for freezing.

COURGETTE FRITTERS WITH MINTY DIP

Courgette is probably my favourite veg, so I do use them a lot in my cooking. This recipe tastes so fresh and I really love it. It's perfect for a lunch served with a little salad, or as a snack on its own with the mint dip, and would be a perfect lunchbox addition too.

 V

Makes: 8 fritters
Prep time: 10 minutes
Cook time: 20 minutes

1 large courgette (about 300g)
40g mature cheddar cheese, coarsely grated
6 spring onions, trimmed and finely chopped
grated zest of ½ lemon
6 tbsp wholemeal self-raising flour
1 large free-range egg
½ tsp garam masala
olive oil, for frying
rocket or salad leaves to serve (optional)

FOR THE MINTY DIP
4 sprigs of mint, leaves picked
  and very finely chopped
150g natural or Greek yoghurt
juice of ½ lemon
1 tbsp mango chutney (optional)

1. Grate the courgettes onto a board. Squeeze handfuls of the grated courgette into a bowl and squidge out as much moisture as possible. Get rid of the liquid then add the courgettes, cheddar, spring onions and lemon zest to a bowl. Give it a mix then add in the flour, egg, garam masala. Mix to combine.

2. Pre-heat a large non-stick frying pan on medium heat, add a little olive oil. Once the oil is hot, dollop in 4 heaped spoonfuls of the mix (you need to make 8 in total) and fry for 8–10 minutes, flipping the fritter every 2 minutes to cook both sides until golden and cooked through.

3. Repeat with the other 4 spoonfuls. Leave to cool and firm up for a few minutes on a little kitchen roll to drain excess oil, and then serve.

4. Quickly mix the chopped mint, yoghurt and lemon juice and/or mango chutney (if using), serve alongside (or dolloped on top of the fritters) and serve.

For babies and young children: Fritters work really well for babies who have experienced quite a few different textures. You can chop them into little finger foods to offer to younger children for self-feeding.

ONE-POT CHEESY GREENS PASTA

This refreshing pasta dish is really easy to pop together and easy to adapt, too. You can use whatever greens you have, adjusting the cooking time accordingly. It also works at room temperature for lunch the next day, and makes a great packed-lunch! The pangrattato topping on page 203 goes so well with this meal: it adds extra crunch, texture and nutrients.

Serves: 4
Prep time: 10 minutes
Cook time: 12 minutes

300g pasta (penne or fusilli,
    or any pasta shape you have)
200g frozen peas
200g green beans, trimmed and cut into
    3cm lengths (leave some full length for
    younger babies to munch on)
¼ garlic clove, peeled and finely grated
finely grated zest and juice of 1 lemon
2 tbsp extra-virgin olive oil
100g grated mozzarella
handful basil leaves, roughly chopped,
    to serve

1. Cook the pasta in boiling water for 10 minutes, adding the peas and green beans halfway through, until the pasta is tender and the vegetables are cooked.
2. Meanwhile, mix the garlic, half the lemon juice and the olive oil together and season if you want to. Just before draining the pasta and vegetables, add 4 tablespoons of the cooking water to the oil mixture.
3. Drain the pasta and vegetables then tip back into the pan, adding the garlic, lemon and oil mixture and stir to combine over a medium heat for 1 minute.
4. Stir through the mozzarella, add the remaining lemon juice and zest, stir through some basil then serve sprinkled with the crispy pangrattato topping (if using) and extra basil leaves if you fancy.

For babies and young children: You can mash the pasta up a little or offer it as a finger food. Leave off the basil leaves.

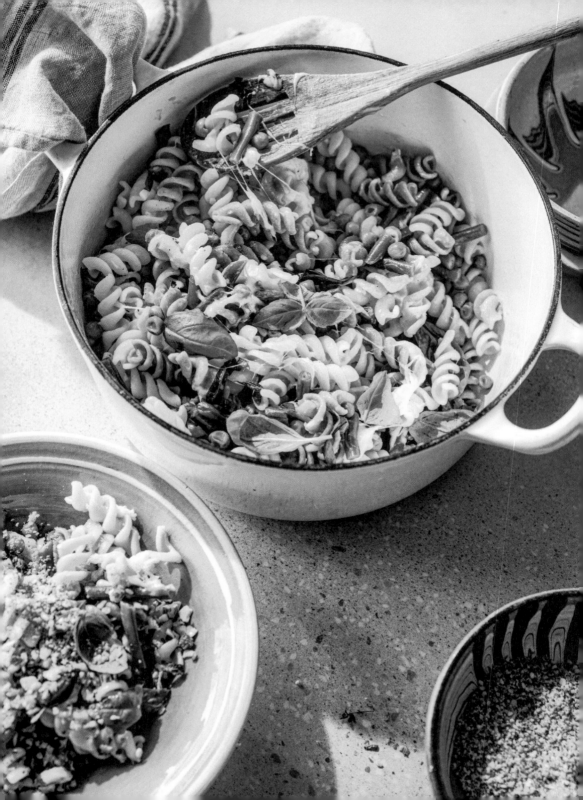

LEFTOVER VEG SOUP

When you have leftover veggies and you don't know what to do with them, here is your answer. This is a super easy, versatile and delicious soup.

Serves: 4–6
Prep time: 10 minutes
Cook time: 40 minutes

1 clove of garlic, peeled and roughly chopped
1 carrot, peeled and roughly chopped (optional)
1 large white or red onion, peeled and roughly chopped
½ tbsp cumin seeds
300g of leftover veg, e.g. courgette, parsnip, fennel bulb, roughly chopped.
1 sweet or normal potato (approx 300g), chopped into 3cm chunks
1 litre of low-salt veg stock or water
400g tin chickpeas, drained

1. To a large pan, add a little oil, on a medium heat. Then add the garlic, carrot and onion.
2. Cook for 10–15 minutes or until soft and a little golden, stirring occasionally. Then add the cumin seeds and cook for another few minutes.
3. Add the leftover vegetables and cook for 5 minutes, then add the potato, water or stock, and continue cooking for 15–20 minutes (or until the potato is cooked).
4. Once the potato is cooked you can blend it up, then add the chickpeas, or you can add the chickpeas and blend to a smooth soup. It's up to you!
5. Serve, and season the adults' to taste if you like.

For babies and young children: Use veggie sticks or sticks of bread to encourage self-feeding with soup.

STUFFED CALZONE PITTAS

These pitta pockets were an idea I had halfway through creating the recipes for this book. I always do pitta pizzas with the tomato sauce on the top, but wanted to try these with a non-cook, easy filling. They are such a nice quick lunch option for the whole family.

Makes: 4 stuffed pittas + leftover pizza filling
Prep time: 10 minutes
Cook time: 20 minutes

4 wholemeal pitta breads
1 small tin of sweetcorn, drained
100g/1 large handful of diced fresh tomatoes
½ a red pepper, diced
100g mushrooms, diced
300g passata sauce
60g grated mozzarella
½ tbsp oregano
optional extra pizza toppings: shredded chicken, lentils, chopped ham, chopped olives, anchovies, tuna, pineapple

1. Add all ingredients (minus the pitta breads) to a bowl and mix well.
2. Use a knife to carefully open the pitta, lengthways across the side.
3. Stuff the mixture into the inside of the pitta bread – use a spoon to squash plenty in, and top with a little extra cheese, if you wish.
4. Pop on a lined baking tray, cover with a layer of tin foil and bake in oven for 15–20 minutes, until warm and a little crisp (take the tin foil off for the last 5 minutes if you'd like to crisp up the pitta).
5. Serve with a little side salad.

For babies and young children:
They might find this easier to dissect and eat the middle with a spoon, or tear the pitta and use it as a dip. For very young babies, even the well-chopped veggies might be a bit of a tricky texture for them, so you could always give the filling a blend.

CREAMY MUSHROOM PANCAKES

Mushrooms are always a hit in our house and so are pancakes, so this one was bound to be a winner! This recipe takes a little time over the hob, but it's well worth it. Spelt has a mild nutty flavour that works brilliantly with earthy mushrooms and spinach – if you prefer, you can substitute with plain flour instead. This is a lovely one for lunch or dinner too.

Batter makes: 5 large pancakes
Prep time: 10 minutes
Cook time: 25–30 minutes

FOR THE PANCAKE BATTER
120g spelt or plain flour
2 medium free-range eggs
220ml milk of choice
knob of butter or drizzle of oil, for frying

FOR THE FILLING
knob of butter or 1 tbsp olive oil
400g chestnut mushrooms, sliced
2 spring onions, trimmed and thinly sliced
100g spinach, washed and chopped or torn
1 garlic clove, peeled and crushed/chopped
2 sprigs of thyme, leaves picked
dollop or drizzle of something creamy (e.g., double cream, crème fraîche, mascarpone, cream cheese or dairy-free alternative) (optional)

1. To make the batter, put all the ingredients into a measuring jug, then whizz with a stick blender or whisk with a hand whisk until completely smooth – it should be quite thin, the texture of single cream. Leave to rest while you make the filling.
2. Heat a large frying pan over a high heat and add the butter or oil. Once the butter is sizzling or the oil shimmers, add the mushrooms to the pan, spread them out as much as you can and cook for 2–3 minutes with minimal stirring. Once the water they release has evaporated and they are cooking, stir to gently flip them over and cook the other side, then add the spring onions and cook for 2–3 minutes without much stirring.
3. Add the spinach to the pan and let it wilt slightly before stirring it through the mushrooms and onions. Add the garlic and thyme leaves and let everything cook for 2 minutes. Stir through the cream or crème fraîche, if using, then set aside somewhere warm.
4. To make the pancakes, turn the heat to medium-high, add the butter or oil and wipe it round the pan a little with a brush or some kitchen paper. Once the pan is hot, pour in just enough mixture to coat the pan in a thin layer when you swirl it around.
5. Once it's evenly coated, return to the heat and cook for 2–3 minutes, until the sides are crisp and the underside is golden.
6. Flip it over, return to the heat and cook for another 30 seconds–1 minute, until the underside has golden spots.

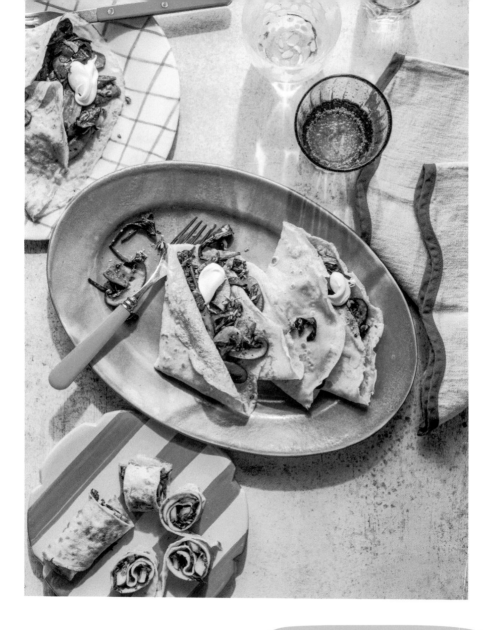

7. Slide the pancake onto a warm plate and repeat until you have made all the pancakes.
8. Bring the filling back to a sizzle quickly on the hob, then fill the pancakes – either in the middle with the pancakes folded over, or spread a thin layer of filling over the whole pancake then roll up and cut into slices. Serve immediately.

For babies and young children: These can be rolled up tightly and chopped into little rings for baby to self-feed, or you could blend the ingredients in the middle and spread it on a pancake before chopping into strips – whichever you think your baby needs for their skill development.

Dinner

TOMATO AND SARDINE SAUCE

This is such a simple, quick recipe made with just a few store-cupboard ingredients. You can adapt it as you wish – adding extra flavours, using less sardines, adding some cheese…it's so easy to tweak. The sardines are a great source of omega-3 fatty acids, and tinned ones have soft bones which contain high levels of calcium, so are good options to include in a sauce for the whole family, and especially great for growing kids! This recipe makes a big batch and is freezable, so it's perfect to make in advance.

Makes: about 800g sauce
Prep time: 5 minutes
Cook time: 10–15 minutes

2 x 120g tins sardines in olive oil
2 large garlic cloves, peeled and crushed
2 x 400g tins chopped tomatoes
10g parsley or chives, finely chopped
cooked pasta or gnocchi, to serve

1. Heat a large sauté or frying pan over a medium heat and tip in the sardines and garlic.
2. Allow them to warm through, breaking up the sardines – the garlic will soften but don't allow it to colour at all.
3. Add the tomatoes, bring to a simmer and cook for 8–10 minutes, stirring often, until reduced and thick.
4. Stir through the herbs, then serve with cooked pasta or gnocchi, or freeze in portions for another day.

For babies and young children: This is fine as it is, but if you want a smoother sauce you can always give it a little mash or add a splash of water and blend down before offering to babies.

COVER ALL CURRY

Curries are a go-to for many families, but can be tricky if your kids aren't familiar with hotter, spicier flavours. This curry is a perfect ease-in – it's easy to adapt the heat (if you want more spice, add more), but it's also simple, has a lovely flavour and contains veggies that children usually love! You can easily vary the veggies, of course. This one was a winner with Raffy and has become a firm favourite.

Serves: 4
Prep time: 10 minutes
Cook time: 25–30 minutes

1 tbsp vegetable oil
1 white onion, peeled and thinly sliced
2 garlic cloves, peeled and finely
    chopped or crushed
handful of coriander, stalks finely chopped
    and leaves reserved for the top,
    or ½ tbsp dried coriander
1 carrot, peeled and cut into thin rounds
300g butternut squash, peeled, deseeded
    and cut into 2cm chunks
½–1 tbsp mild curry powder
400ml tin coconut milk
400g tin chickpeas, drained
100g mangetout, roughly chopped into thirds
200ml hot water

TO SERVE
cooked basmati rice
dairy-free or natural yoghurt
lime wedges

1. Heat the oil in a large frying pan (or wok) over a medium heat, add the onion, garlic, coriander stalks (no tops) and carrot. Cook for 5 minutes, stirring occasionally.
2. Add the butternut squash and mild curry powder and cook, stirring, for another 5 minutes.
3. Add the coconut milk, 200ml of hot water and the chickpeas and cook for 15–20 minutes (until the squash is soft and the sauce reduces a little).
4. Add the mangetout for the final 5 minutes.
5. Serve with rice, yoghurt dolloped on top and the picked coriander leaves (if you fancy) and a squeeze of lime.

For babies and young children: Blend the sauce with the veggies in a separate bowl, or just make sure you chop/mash the chickpeas and veggies really well for toddlers. You also might want to go easier with the curry powder.

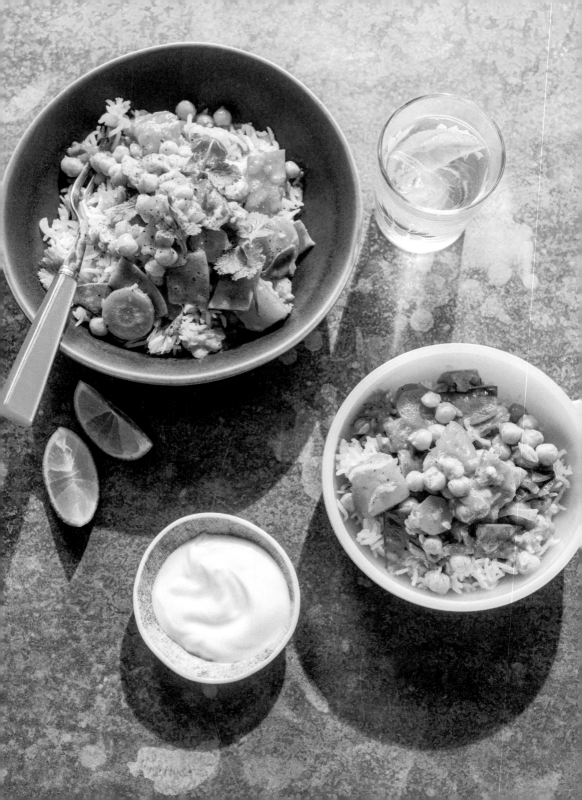

CHICKEN AND ORZO ONE-POT

I love this recipe. It's super refreshing with the lemon, which complements the rest of the ingredients so well, and it's an easy, incredibly comforting crowd-pleaser. Best of all there's minimal washing up!

Serves: 4 with leftovers
Prep time: 10–15 minutes
Cook time: 50 mins

6 bone-in, skin-on chicken thighs
   or 250g Quorn chicken-style pieces
3 leeks, washed, cut into rounds
   and then halved
3 garlic cloves, peeled and crushed
250g orzo
1 litre chicken stock/low-salt stock or water
a little oil
120g frozen peas
lemon juice, to taste
basil leaves, to serve

1. Preheat the oven to 200°C/180°C fan. Place a large, shallow oven- and flame-proof pan over a medium-high heat and add the chicken thighs, skin-side down.
2. Fry for 5–6 minutes, until the skin is deep golden and crisp, then flip them over and fry the other side for a minute. Transfer to a plate and discard some of the fat in the pan if you want to.
3. Add a little oil to the pan first if you're using Quorn rather than chicken, then add the leeks and fry, stirring often, for 5–10 minutes until softened. Add the garlic and fry, stirring constantly, for 2 minutes, then add the orzo and stir it evenly through the leeks.
4. Pour in the stock or water, bring to a simmer, then nestle the chicken thighs into the pan, skin-side up. If using Quorn, simply add it to the pan and give it a good stir before popping it into the oven.
5. Transfer to the oven and cook, uncovered, for 40–45 minutes, stirring in the peas for the last 10 minutes.
6. Once everything is cooked, the orzo should still be a little soupy. Divide among bowls and add lemon juice to taste and torn basil leaves.

For babies and young children: Remove any chicken skin. Offer strips of chicken for them to self-feed and chop the cooked veggies nice and small. Give it a good mash if needed before serving.

TURKEY BURGER

I couldn't write a family cookbook without including a burger recipe! I wanted to use a different meat to make a really tasty variation on your average burger. We love to serve with homemade fries or wedges, but this will also go really well with the Parmesan, Carrot and Parsnip Batons on page 220.

Serves: 4–6
Prep time: 10 minutes
Cook time: 10–15 minutes

500g turkey mince
1 large free-range egg
4 spring onions, trimmed and finely chopped
1 tsp dried cumin
1 tsp ground coriander
1 tsp paprika
1 tbsp olive oil

TO SERVE
4–6 wholemeal burger buns
30g cheddar cheese, sliced
1 large tomato, thinly sliced
handful of spinach leaves, washed
    (and chopped for kids)

FOR THE ZESTY MAYO
2 tbsp tomato purée (or ketchup)
3 tbsp yoghurt (or mayonnaise)
grated zest and juice of ½ a lime

1. Put the mince, egg, spring onions and spices in a bowl, mix well and squish together. Form the mixture into 4 patties, 2 smaller and 2 larger (8–9cm wide, 1.5cm thick).
2. Heat the oil in a large frying pan over a medium heat. Add the patties (or a couple if only cooking for a few) and cook for 6 minutes on each side, turning them every 3 minutes to get a good colour.
3. Meanwhile, halve and toast the buns.
4. Make a quick tomato mayo. Mix the tomato purée and mayo in a bowl with a squeeze of lime juice and touch of zest.
5. Once the burgers are cooked through, transfer to a plate lined with kitchen paper to drain any excess oil.
6. Serve the buns filled with a little lime ketchup, the cooked burger, a little cheese, sliced tomato and spinach.

For babies and young children: Offer the burger cut in sticks for younger babies, or make mini burgers for them to dissect, served with tomato purée and yoghurt.

SPEEDY

SWEET POTATO AND LENTIL DHAL

This comforting and delicious dinner is easy to double up so you have a batch ready to freeze. It's quick to make, flavourful and packed full of nutrients. Serve with rice or couscous, with bread for dipping (see the Coconut Flatbread recipe on page 221).

Serves: 4, plus plenty of leftovers
Prep time: 15 minutes
Cook: 25–30 minutes

1 tbsp sunflower oil
1 onion, peeled and finely diced
2 garlic cloves, peeled and crushed
3cm piece of root ginger, peeled and grated
½–1 tbsp mild curry powder, to taste
200g passata
200g dried red lentils
2 medium sweet potatoes, peeled and
    cut into 2cm chunks
juice of ½–1 lemon, to taste

TO SERVE
10g fresh mint, leaves well chopped
dairy-free or natural yoghurt (optional)
black onion or sesame seeds

1. Heat the oil in a large, lidded saucepan over a medium-high heat, add the onion and fry for 5 minutes, until softened and beginning to colour.
2. Add the garlic, ginger and curry powder and fry for 2 minutes, stirring, until fragrant. Then add the passata, lentils, sweet potatoes and 800ml water.
3. Bring everything to a simmer, cover and cook for 10 minutes over a low-medium heat, then remove the lid and simmer for a further 10 minutes, until the sweet potato is tender and the dhal has thickened.
4. Add lemon juice to taste, then divide among bowls, scatter with the mint, drizzle with a little yoghurt (if using) and finish with a sprinkling of black onion or sesame seeds.

For babies and young children:
Leave out the mint garnish.

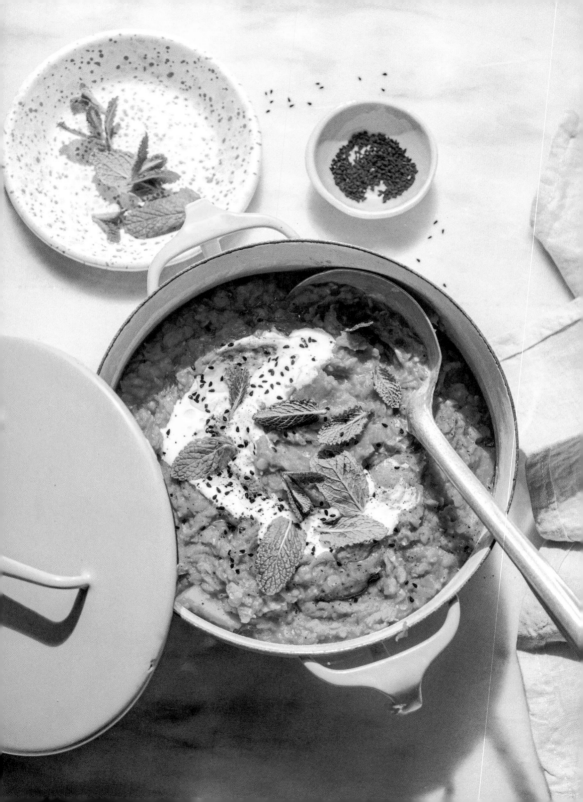

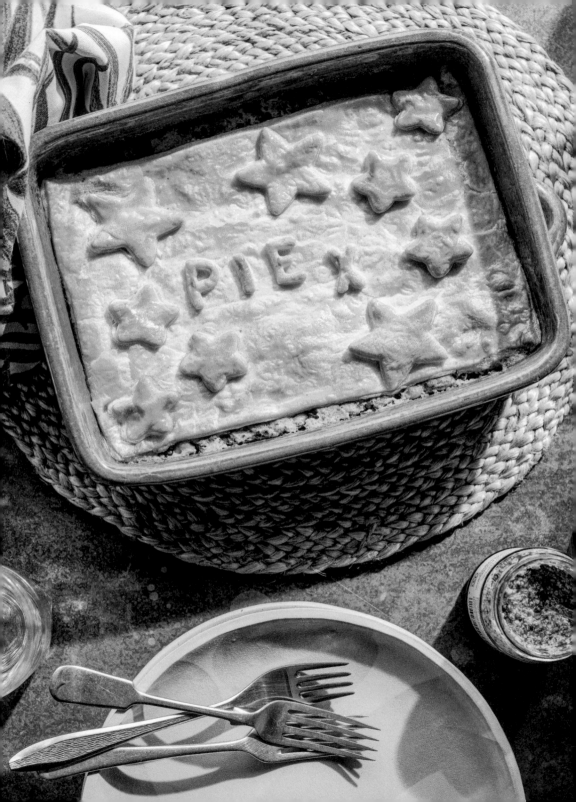

GREEN VEG AND LENTIL PIE

Making a pie may feel like a lot of effort, but this one is easy to put together and tastes delicious. You can make your own pastry (see page 218) or use shop-bought puff. This warming, nutritious option makes a meal in itself, but is also nice served with potatoes and beans on the side. It's super quick to prep!

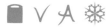

Serves: 4
Prep time: 10 minutes
Cook time: 40–50 minutes

300g frozen green vegetables (I used a mix of peas, broad and green beans, or spinach, peas and broccoli)
400g tin black or green lentils, drained and rinsed
220–250g crème fraîche (or dairy free alt)
2 tbsp grainy mustard
1 garlic clove, peeled and crushed
large pinch of smoked paprika
large pinch of ground cumin
½ x 320g sheet ready-rolled puff pastry, cut to fit your pie dish
1 medium free-range egg, beaten (optional – works fine without, but won't have a glazed top)

1. Preheat the oven to 200°C/180°C fan. Mix the frozen vegetables with the lentils in a small pie or gratin dish.
2. Mix the crème fraîche, mustard, garlic and spices together, then stir it through the veg and lentils.
3. Lay the pastry over the top, pressing it into the edges, then cut a steam hole in the centre.
4. Brush all over with beaten egg (if using) then place on a baking tray and bake in the oven for 40–50 minutes, until the pastry is deep golden and crisp all over, and the filling is bubbling underneath.
5. Remove from the oven and allow to stand for 2–3 minutes before serving.

For babies and young children: Offer just the insides, mashed well and a few strips of the pastry separately.

QUORN FAJITAS

My kids love fajitas! The 'pic 'n' mix' options help make mealtime fun and adds autonomy for small hands. Quorn can be a great alternative to chicken, but feel free to use cooked chicken instead. This recipe looks complex but it's really not – it's four separate and very quick elements that combine together so nicely.

This spice mix is one of my favourites as it's delicious and doesn't have the salt and sugar you find in shop-bought fajita spice mixes – it lasts a while too, so you can use it to make a few more meals!

 ∨ ⅄

Serves: 4, plus extra spice mix
Prep time: 10 minutes
Cook time: 25 minutes

FOR THE BLACK BEANS
splash of olive oil
1 garlic clove, peeled and thinly sliced
1 tsp smoked paprika
400g tin black beans (not drained!)

FOR THE SPICE MIX
4 tbsp smoked paprika
4 tbsp ground cumin
2 tbsp ground coriander
2 tbsp garlic powder/granules
2 tbsp dried oregano

FOR THE QUORN FILLING
350g frozen Quorn pieces
drizzle of olive oil

FOR THE GUACAMOLE
2 ripe avocados, destoned and mashed
handful of cherry tomatoes (about 80g), finely chopped
handful of coriander, finely chopped (optional)
juice of 1 lime, plus ½ cut into wedges for serving
1 tbsp olive oil
1 red chilli, deseeded and finely diced (optional)

TO SERVE
8 small wholemeal tortilla wraps
200g thick Greek yoghurt, dairy-free alternative or soured cream
50g cheddar cheese (optional)
salad leaves (shredded little gem or baby spinach leaves work well)

1. Start by making the guacamole, mix and mash all the ingredients into a large bowl and leave to the side.
2. Put a saucepan on a medium/high heat with a splash of oil and add the garlic and smoked paprika – cook for a few minutes, then add the black beans (juice and all) and cook for 8–10 mins, stirring occasionally until thickened but reduced by half. You can mash it a little so it is more like a paste, or keep it chunky. Turn off and cover to one side until serving.
3. Meanwhile mix the spices in a small bowl or glass jar. Leave to one side.
4. Add a little oil to a medium frying pan and add the Quorn and 1 tablespoon of spice mix. Cook for a few minutes then add a couple of splashes of water, moving around the pan to defrost and cook. Continue cooking for another 8 minutes.
5. Warm the tortillas in the oven or pop them in the microwave for 30 seconds.
6. Serve everything up in bowls on the table and let your family dig in!

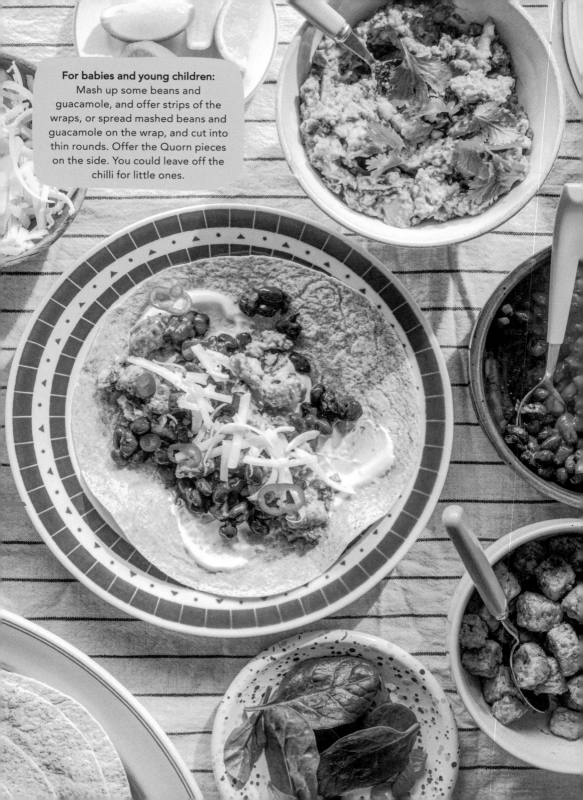

For babies and young children:
Mash up some beans and guacamole, and offer strips of the wraps, or spread mashed beans and guacamole on the wrap, and cut into thin rounds. Offer the Quorn pieces on the side. You could leave off the chilli for little ones.

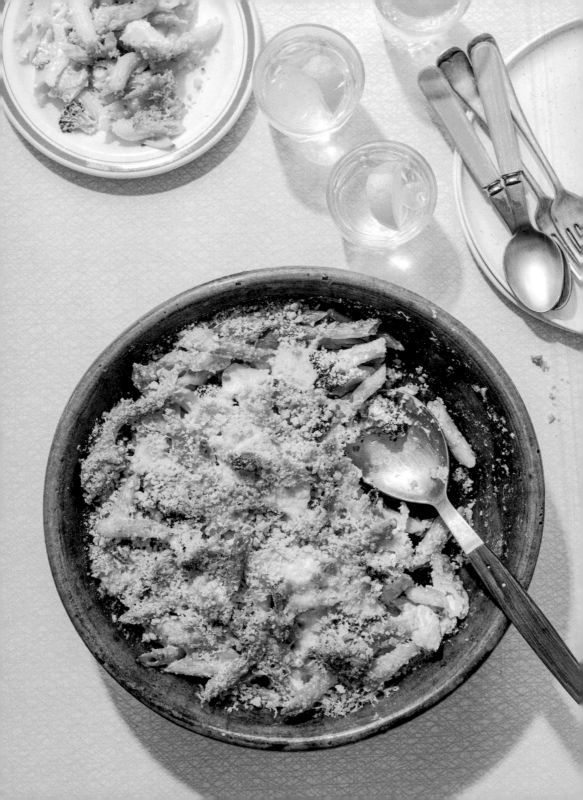

BROCCOLI AND FISH PIESTER BAKE

This is like a mash-up between a fish pie and a pasta bake, hence the name 'piester bake'. We love this in our house and it's an easy one to cook, with refreshing and fragrant flavours from the lemon and nutmeg.

Serves: 4
Prep time: 15 minutes
Cook time: 25–30 minutes

250g any pasta shape
200g broccoli, cut into bite-sized pieces
300g crème fraîche
¼ tsp ground nutmeg
juice and zest of 1 lemon
250g fish (I use a mix of cod and salmon),
   cut into 2cm chunks
50g dried or fresh breadcrumbs
50g cheddar cheese, grated, or sprinkling
   of nutritional yeast

1. Preheat the oven to 200°C/180°C fan.
2. Cook the pasta in boiling water for 2 minutes less than stated on the packet instructions, until it's just al dente (add the broccoli to the pan as well).
3. Mix the crème fraîche, nutmeg and lemon juice together in a bowl.
4. When the pasta is cooked, drain it well – reserving a spoonful of the cooking water – then toss the pasta together with the fish in an ovenproof pan or dish.
5. Pour over the crème fraîche mixture and add the reserved pasta water, then stir everything together until well coated.
6. Scatter over the breadcrumbs and cheddar or nutritional yeast, then bake in the oven for 20–25 minutes.
7. Remove from the oven and allow to stand for 2 minutes, then serve.

For babies and young children: Give it all a little mash with a fork or simply offer sticks of pasta, broccoli and salmon.

MEXICAN TOMATO SOUP

This is a very versatile tomato soup and makes loads of leftovers. There are lots of options for garnishes – if you put a range of them out on the table, kids will love to help themselves and top their soup how they like it.

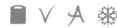

Makes: about 2 litres
Prep time: 15 minutes
Cook time: 20 minutes

2 tbsp olive oil
1 red onion, peeled and sliced
2 garlic cloves, peeled and crushed
2 tsp ground cumin
2 tsp ground coriander
½ tsp ground cinnamon
¼ tsp ground allspice
3 x 400g tins chopped tomatoes
800ml vegetable stock (low- or no-salt stock for young children) or water
2 x 400g tins kidney beans, drained and rinsed

OPTIONAL GARNISHES
Greek yoghurt or soured cream
    (or dairy-free yoghurt)
toasted tortilla wraps, broken-up into pieces
pumpkin seeds
coriander sprigs
ripe avocado, finely diced
fresh chillies, chopped
pickled jalapenos

1. Heat the oil in a large saucepan over a medium-high heat, add the onion and fry for 5 minutes, stirring often, until softened and slightly coloured. Reduce the heat to medium, add the garlic and spices and stir for 2 minutes, until really fragrant.
2. Add the tomatoes with the stock or water. Bring everything to a simmer, then cook for 15 minutes, until the liquid has thickened slightly.
3. Blitz the soup with a stick blender until smooth, then stir in the kidney beans, return to a simmer and cook for another 5 minutes.
4. Ladle into bowls and garnish with your choice of ingredients. Leftovers can be frozen or will keep in the fridge for up to 3 days.

For babies and young children: Be careful with toppings. Offer the soup with mashed or blended kidney beans to young babies, and stir in some yoghurt and have some advocado on the side. The seeds and wraps may be a choking hazard, so leave these for the older kids in the family.

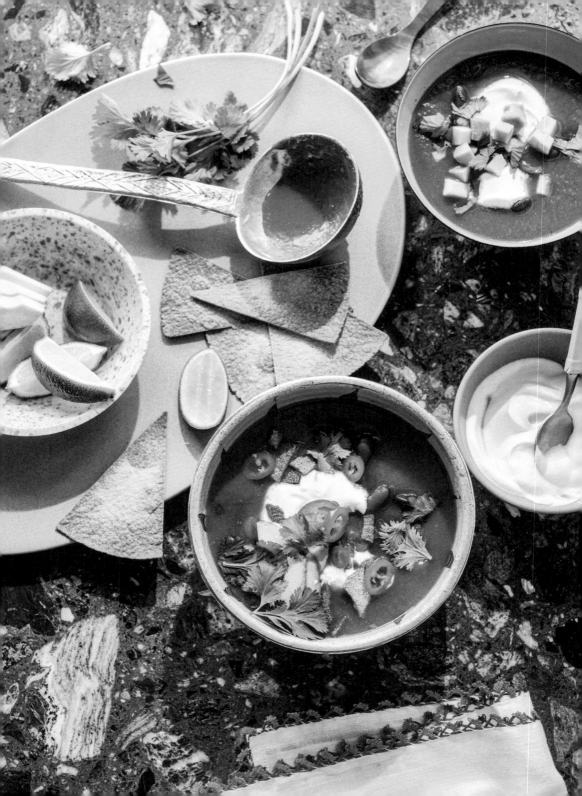

CREAMY TOMATO AND SPINACH GNOCCHI

I adore gnocchi as a variation for pasta. This recipe uses fresh tomatoes, but you can easily swap them for tinned, for ease and speed. It's a bit different for an evening meal, I love whipping this out for the kids as it's a firm favourite!

Serves: 4
Prep time: 20 minutes
Cook time: 15–20 minutes

olive oil, for frying
1 red onion, peeled and finely diced
2 garlic cloves, peeled and thinly
   sliced or crushed
500g fresh cherry tomatoes
   (or 400g tin chopped tomatoes)
120g spinach, washed and well chopped
80g cream cheese or dairy-free alternative
400g pack of fresh gnocchi
1 x can cannellini beans, drained and
   rinsed
dried chilli flakes, to serve (optional,
   for adults)
100ml water

1. Heat a drizzle of oil in a frying pan over a medium heat. Add the onion and fry for a few minutes, stirring often and not allowing it to colour, until soft. Add the garlic and fry for 2 minutes more, then add the tomatoes with 100ml water (or tinned tomatoes instead, if using, and skip to step 3).

2. Increase the heat slightly and cook for 8 minutes, stirring often. Once the tomatoes start to soften, use a wooden spoon to gently squash them so they release their juices.

3. Once the tomatoes are collapsing and soft, add the spinach to the pan and allow it to wilt. Stir through the cream cheese, then set aside.

4. Cook the gnocchi and beans according to the gnocchi packet instructions (the beans just need to heat through for a couple of minutes), then just before draining the gnocchi transfer a ladle of the cooking water to the sauce.

5. Drain the gnocchi and beans, then stir through the sauce over a low heat for 2 minutes, until everything is well coated. Serve immediately (adults might like a sprinkling of dried chilli flakes).

For babies and young children: Gnocchi can be a choking hazard, so slice them up once cooked for younger kids. For babies, leave them out and just serve the sauce with pasta!

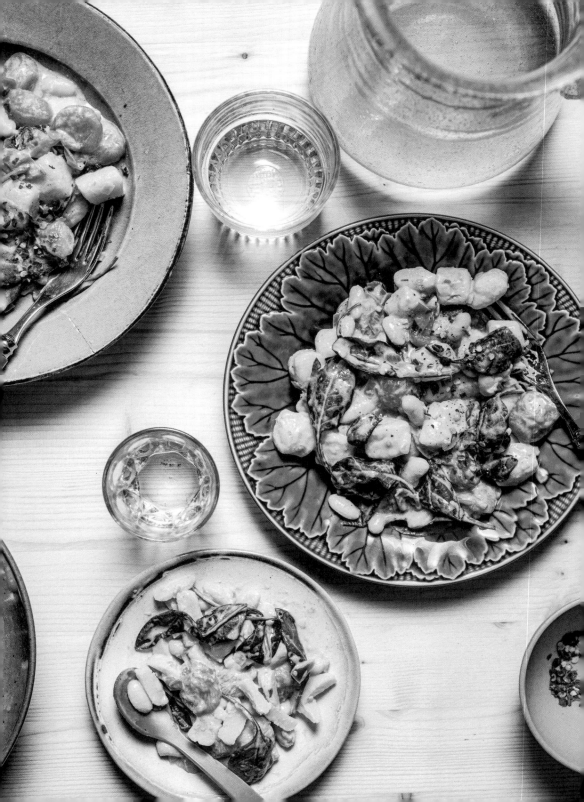

THAI-STYLE POT-ROAST CAULIFLOWER

If you're looking for a more 'fancy' vegetarian centrepiece, then this is the one for you. The cauliflower, with a mild coconutty Thai-style sauce, will be a hit with everyone. It works so well with rice or noodles, and you can use the leftover sauce to create some lovely extra recipes. The flavours are absolutely delicious.

Serves: 4, with some sauce leftovers
Prep time: 25 minutes
Cook time: 1 hour 10 minutes

1 small onion, peeled and roughly chopped
3 garlic cloves, peeled and roughly chopped
3cm piece of root ginger, peeled and sliced
2 lemongrass stalks, outer layers discarded,
     stalks roughly chopped
½ x 1g jar dried makrut lime leaves
1 tsp ground cumin
1–2 tsp mild chilli powder (optional)
finely grated zest and juice of 1 lime
50g coriander, leaves and stalks
     roughly chopped
3 tbsp coconut oil or sunflower oil
2 x 400g tins coconut milk
800ml vegetable stock (no- or low-salt)
     or water
1 cinnamon stick
1 large cauliflower, outer leaves removed

TO SERVE
50g roasted unsalted peanuts,
     finely chopped (optional)
cooked noodles or rice
lime wedges

Cook's tip: You need a decent amount of sauce to properly cook the cauliflower, so you may end up with some leftover, which can make a variety of different meals. You can stir cooked chicken or firm tofu through it to make another meal, or add some noodles and mushrooms to make a noodle soup. The possibilities are endless!

1. Preheat the oven to 180°C/160°C fan. Put the onion, garlic, ginger, lemongrass, half the lime leaves, cumin, chilli powder (if using), lime zest and coriander stalks into a small food processor with 2 tablespoons of water. Blitz until you have a smooth paste.

2. Heat the oil in a large oven- and flame-proof lidded casserole dish (deep enough to contain the whole cauliflower) over a medium-high heat. Add the paste and fry for 5–6 minutes, stirring constantly, until the paste is fragrant and darker in colour.

3. Add the coconut milk and stock with the rest of the lime leaves and cinnamon, and bring to a simmer. Add the cauliflower, put the lid on and transfer to the oven. Cook for 50 minutes, basting with the sauce once or twice.

4. After 50 minutes remove the lid, baste again. Increase the oven temperature to 200°C/180°C fan. Roast for a further 10–15 minutes, until the top of the cauliflower is lightly browned.

5. Remove from the oven, scatter over the coriander leaves and peanuts (if using). Squeeze in the lime and season if you like (remove small children's portions first). Cut the cauliflower into portions and divide among bowls with rice or noodles, ladle over plenty of sauce, and serve with extra lime wedges for squeezing.

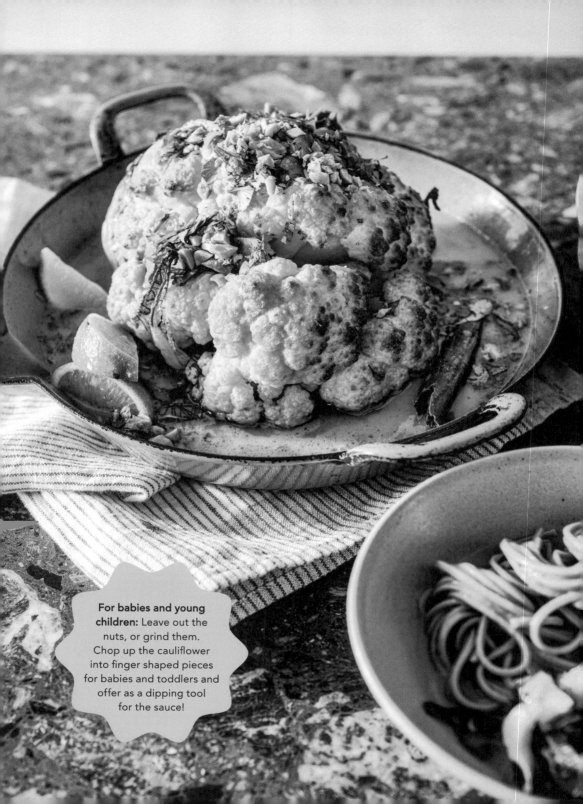

For babies and young children: Leave out the nuts, or grind them. Chop up the cauliflower into finger shaped pieces for babies and toddlers and offer as a dipping tool for the sauce!

3-WAY PASTA SAUCE

A basic pasta sauce recipe is pretty much essential for every family, right? With this one I wanted to offer multiple options: one is a simple, covers-everything recipe, which packs plenty of flavour and veg; one is an 'added extras' recipe that's veggie-based but with more texture and nutrients; and finally there's a version for those who like it meaty! They are also all perfect options for making in bulk and freezing in portions, ideal for when you need a quick pasta option in the evenings!

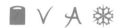

Makes:
Simple tomato sauce – about 600g
Extra veggie sauce – about 1 kilo (portioned up into 500g batches) (serves 4–6)
Meaty sauce – about 1 kilo
Prep time: 10 minutes
Cook time: variable

NOTE: If you don't have a food processor you will need to keep the veg whole, and coarsely grate it or use a mini chopper.

SIMPLE TOMATO SAUCE
1 red or white onion, peeled
    and roughly chopped
2 medium carrots, peeled
    and roughly chopped
olive oil, for frying
1 garlic clove, peeled and finely chopped
½ tbsp dried mixed herbs or a handful of fresh
basil, stalks finely chopped, leaves roughly
    chopped (saving some for later)
400g tin chopped tomatoes
2 tbsp tomato purée

FOR THE EXTRA VEGGIE VERSION
150g chestnut mushrooms, halved
1 red pepper, deseeded and roughly chopped
400g tin cooked lentils, drained

TO MAKE IT MEATY
400g good-quality beef mince

1. If you have a food processor you can save yourself a lot of time here. Pop the onion and carrots into the food processor and pulse to chop, making sure they don't go all mushy. You want them to look as they would if you chopped them really well by hand. If you don't have a food processor, grate the veggies instead.
2. Put a large ragu-type pan onto a medium heat, with a splash of oil. After a few minutes add the onion, carrots, garlic, dried herbs and basil, if using fresh basil (stalks only). Cook for 5 minutes stirring occasionally. If you're keeping the sauce simple, now skip to step 5.
3. **For the extra veggie version**, pulse the mushrooms and pepper in a food processor to cut them into really small pieces. Add to the pan on a medium heat, stirring to combine the vegetables for around 8 minutes.

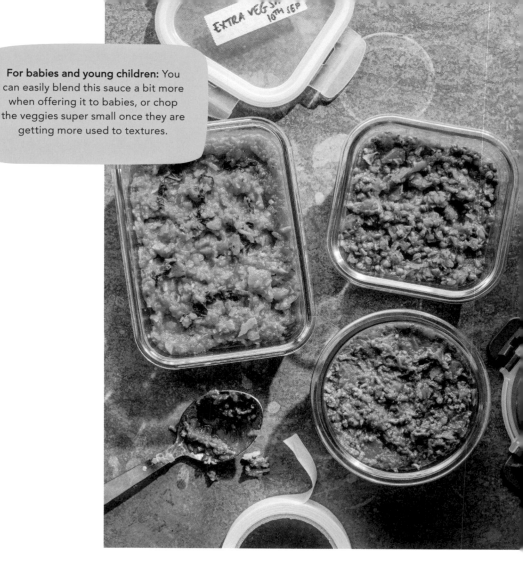

For babies and young children: You can easily blend this sauce a bit more when offering it to babies, or chop the veggies super small once they are getting more used to textures.

4. **For the meaty version**: once the veg is looking all lovely and golden, push to one side, add another splash of oil and add the mince. Cook for 5 minutes, combining the veggies with the meat after a few minutes to mix it all together.

5. Now it's time to add the tomato purée, stir in with the veg (and meat, if using), then add the tinned tomatoes, fill the can halfway with hot water and add, stirring well.

6. Simmer now for 10–15 minutes until thickened and tasting delicious.

7. **For the extra veggie version**, add the lentils while it is simmering, and stir to combine. Bring to the boil then your sauce is ready!

8. Use straight away, or cool and store in batches in the fridge or freezer. All sauces will keep in the fridge for up to 4 days, or can be frozen for up to 3 months.

BAKED RISOTTO

This delicious 'cheat's' risotto means you don't need to be standing at the hob stirring – baked risottos are a great quick option. I've included topping options here to give this recipe a little mix up, and you can vary these depending on what you've got in the house. We love mushrooms, so that's been a favourite for us. It's great without the extra toppings too – but they do add a little something special.

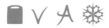

Serves: 2 adults and 2 children with leftovers
Prep time: 10 minutes
Cook time: 30 minutes

50g unsalted butter or 50ml olive oil
1 large onion, peeled and finely chopped
2 medium courgettes, grated
2 garlic cloves, peeled and crushed
250g risotto rice
700ml vegetable stock (made with
   1 low- or no-salt stock cube)
   or water
good squeeze of lemon juice
30g cheddar cheese, plus extra to serve
   (optional)

1. Preheat the oven to 200°C/180°C fan. Melt the butter or heat the oil in an ovenproof frying pan or casserole dish over a medium heat (if you don't have an ovenproof frying pan just use a large normal frying pan and transfer to an oven dish once it's ready for the oven), then add the onion and courgettes and fry for 5–6 minutes, stirring often, until the onion has softened and the courgettes have lost most of their volume.
2. Stir in the garlic and cook for 2 minutes more, then add the rice and stir it through, frying it for a minute or so. Pour in the stock or water, bring to a simmer then stir once more and put in the oven (transferring the contents of the pan to an oven dish if needed). Bake for 20 minutes, stirring halfway through, until the liquid has almost all been absorbed and the rice is tender.

3. Stir through the lemon juice and the cheese if using, and any other flavourings, then serve.

> **Make ahead:** Allow the risotto to cool completely, then portion up into airtight containers and freeze for up to 1 month. Defrost in the fridge thoroughly then reheat in the microwave or on the hob with a splash of water to stop it drying out.

VARIATIONS

MUSHROOM AND THYME
While the risotto is baking, fry 300g roughly sliced chestnut mushrooms in a knob of butter or drizzle of olive oil over a high heat until caramelised and softened. (You can use the frying pan you used for the risotto, to save on washing up, if not using an ovenproof pan.) Add the picked leaves from 3 thyme sprigs for the last couple of minutes, then stir through the risotto once cooked and garnish with a little more fresh thyme.

PRAWN AND TOMATO
While the risotto is baking, fry 150g halved cherry tomatoes with a drizzle of olive oil over a high heat for 3–4 minutes. (You can use the frying pan you used for the risotto, if not using an ovenproof pan.) Once softened, add 200g raw peeled king prawns and fry for a further 2

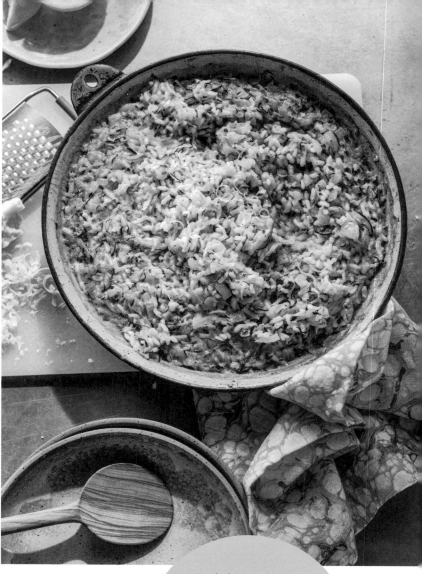

minutes, stirring often, until pink and cooked through. Stir everything through the cooked risotto with the pan juices and garnish with fresh basil.

PEAS AND BEANS

About 8 minutes before the risotto finishes cooking, stir in 250g frozen green vegetables (such as a pea and bean mix, or some peas/green beans/edamame beans) and allow to finish cooking. Garnish with fresh snipped chives.

For babies and young children: Offer the base recipe (made with no-salt stock cube) to little ones, loosening it with some liquid if it's quite thick and sticky. If using the toppings, make sure they are cooked and chopped well, and stirred through and give them a little mash if needed.

PAD THAI

Pad Thai reminds me of dinner with friends in London (pre-kids, when that kind of luxury was more regular!). This recipe is a really delicious one. It's super easy to adapt it for younger kids, and it's so tasty and pretty simple. You can swap the protein, and serve with egg noodles or rice instead!

Serves: 4
Prep time: 10 minutes
Cook time: 15 minutes

150g flat rice noodles
1 tbsp smooth peanut butter
juice of 1 lime
1 tbsp maple syrup or honey
   (leave out for younger babies/toddlers)
3 tbsp olive oil
200g large peeled frozen or cooked
   prawns, sliced chicken breast or firm
   tofu, cut into 2cm chunks
2 garlic cloves, peeled and thinly sliced
1 red onion, peeled and thinly sliced
4 spring onions, trimmed and thinly sliced
handful of sugar snap peas (optional)
2 large free-range eggs, beaten – it works
   without egg, but may be a little drier, so
   may need extra of the peanut butter, honey
   and lime sauce, or a little soy sauce instead
150g beansprouts (optional)
small handful of coriander leaves (optional)

TO SERVE
80g roasted peanuts, ground or chopped
   up (age dependent)
lime wedges
splash of reduced-salt soy sauce (optional)

1. Soak the noodles in a bowl of hot water for 5 minutes to soften, then drain and drizzle with a little oil to stop them sticking. Leave it to one side.

2. To make the sauce, mix the peanut butter, lime juice, maple syrup in a bowl, then add 2–3 tablespoons of hot water to combine. Set aside.

3. Put a large frying pan or wok (if you have one) over a high heat and add 1 tablespoon of the oil. Add the prawns, chicken or tofu (depending on which you're using) and stir-fry for 5 minutes, stirring occasionally. Cook the prawns until pink and hot through, the chicken until browned all over and cooked through, or the tofu until brown on all sides.

4. Transfer to a bowl then add another tablespoon of oil to the pan, then add the garlic, red onion, half the spring onions, the sugar snaps and beansprouts. Cook for 3 minutes until golden and cooked. Pour in the beaten egg, cooked noodles and sauce, and mix and stir to coat.

5. Stir back in the prawns, chicken or tofu then serve topped with crushed nuts, coriander (if using) and lime wedges for squeezing. Serve with soy sauce to taste (leave out for the little ones).

For babies and young children: The mix of different textures might be a bit tricky as it can be tough to coordinate this unless you have a full range of oral motor skills. You can easily offer the noodles, tofu/prawns as finger foods or just those coated in some lime and peanut sauce.

The sauce works well without the honey/maple syrup for babies and toddlers.

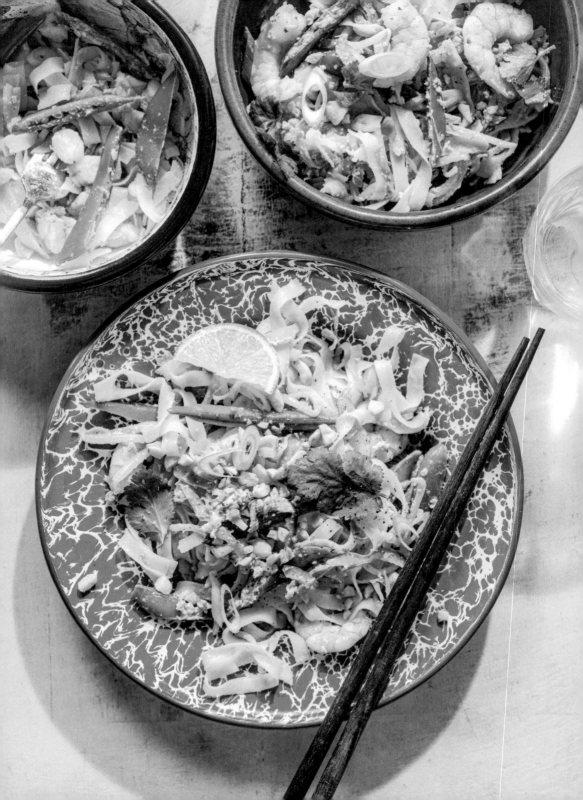

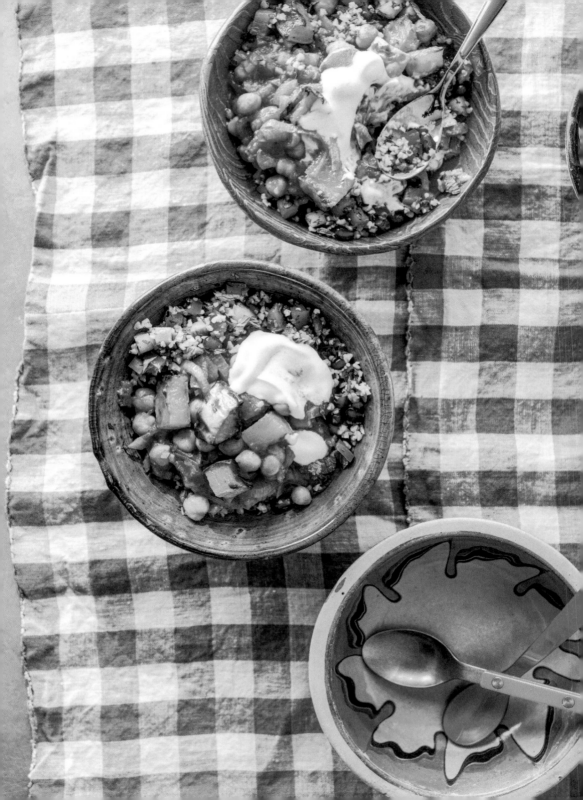

ROAST SQUASH TAGINE

This delicious tagine is one of my favourite recipes in the book. It's a bit more involved, but it's so worth it. Sweet, warming and flavoursome, it's fab alongside the sweet grains on page 133, and great for a dinner party or just Sunday evening at home. This recipe makes plenty, so you'll have some leftovers, which I always love!

Serves: 4–6, plus leftovers will freeze
Prep time: 25 minutes
Cook time: 40 minutes

1 butternut squash, deseeded and cut into
2–3cm chunks (no need to peel)
1 tbsp olive oil, plus extra for drizzling
1 onion, peeled and thinly sliced
3 garlic cloves, peeled and crushed
large pinch of ground ginger
2 tsp ras el hanout
400g tin chopped tomatoes
400g tin chickpeas, drained and rinsed
10 dried apricots, finely chopped

TO SERVE
lemon wedges
pomegranate seeds, coriander (optional)
dairy-free or natural yoghurt (optional)

For babies and young children:
Give the tagine a mash or a blend before serving, especially the chickpeas, and leave out the apricots which could be challenging for younger ones. Also, remove the skin from the squash for babies and older toddlers.

1. Preheat the oven to 200°C/180°C fan. Put the squash on a baking tray, drizzle with a little oil and toss to coat. Roast in the oven for 40 minutes, or until caramelised and soft.
2. Meanwhile, heat the oil in a large, lidded pan over a medium heat, add the onion and fry for 6–8 minutes, stirring often, until softened and beginning to colour. Add the garlic, ginger and ras el hanout and fry, stirring, for another 2–3 minutes, until fragrant.
3. Add the chopped tomatoes, then fill the tin with water and add that too. Stir in the chickpeas and the apricots, then bring everything to a gentle simmer.
4. Put the lid partially on, and simmer gently for 15–20 minutes, stirring occasionally, until the sauce is rich and thickened.
5. Once the sauce has thickened and the squash is ready, gently stir the squash through the sauce and let the tagine stand for 2–3 minutes for the flavours to infuse.
6. Serve with couscous, or the rice dish on page 133, scattered with the pomegranate and herbs, with a dollop of yoghurt if you like.

PORK CASSEROLE WITH ROAST APPLES

This all-in-one casserole lets the oven do all the work for you. The roast apples are a play on apple sauce – they're so delicious you may want to make extra to have with porridge or muesli the next day. This is a really hearty dish and a classic family dinner option. It takes a while to cook, but just 5 minutes to prep, leaving you time to get on with the rest of your to-do list!

Serves: 4 with leftovers
Prep time: 5 minutes
Cook time: 2 hours 30 minutes

500g diced pork shoulder
2 tbsp plain flour
25g unsalted butter
1 onion, peeled and thinly sliced
3 sprigs of rosemary, plus extra chopped rosemary to serve
2 leeks, washed and sliced into rings
500ml chicken stock, low salt preferably
1–2 tbsp wholegrain mustard, to taste
2 eating apples (I used jazz – you need something crunchy), halved
2 tbsp single cream or dairy-free alternative
lemon juice, to taste
baked potatoes, to serve (you can bake them in the oven for 1 hour at the lower heat, then the final 30 minutes at the higher heat)

1. Preheat the oven to 170°C/150°C fan. Toss the pork in the flour, then put in a lidded oven- and flame-proof casserole dish with all the ingredients up to and including the mustard. Bring to a simmer on the hob, then cover and transfer to the oven. Cook for 2 hours.
2. After 2 hours, remove from the oven, take off the lid and give it a stir. It won't look very appealing, but don't worry! Turn the oven temperature up to 200°C/180°C fan and lay the apples out on a baking tray.
3. Return the casserole dish to the oven uncovered, with the apples on the shelf above, and bake for another 30 minutes.
4. After this time the casserole should be reduced to a good saucy texture – if you'd like it a bit thicker, simmer it on the hob for 2–3 minutes. Stir through the cream and lemon juice to taste.
5. Serve the casserole topped with the apples, with baked potatoes, scattered with some extra chopped rosemary.

For babies and young children: Mash the potato with some of the baked apple and sauce. Leave off the potato skin and rosemary.

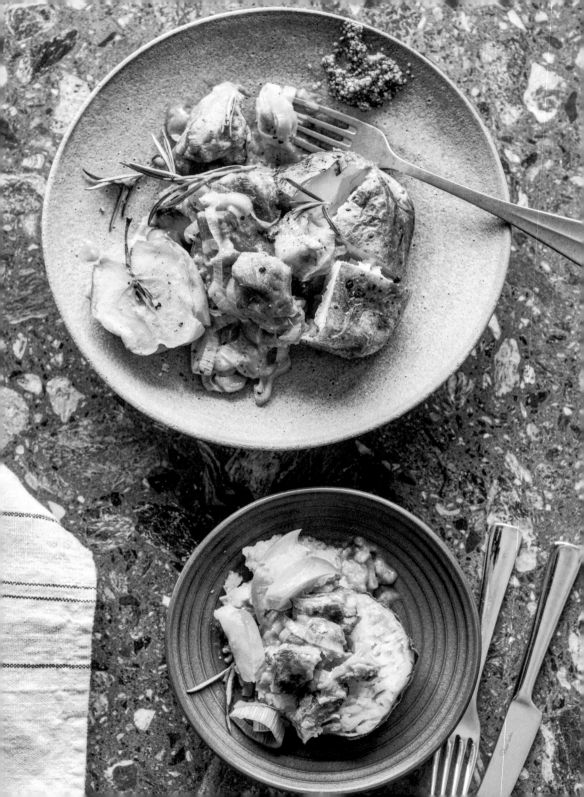

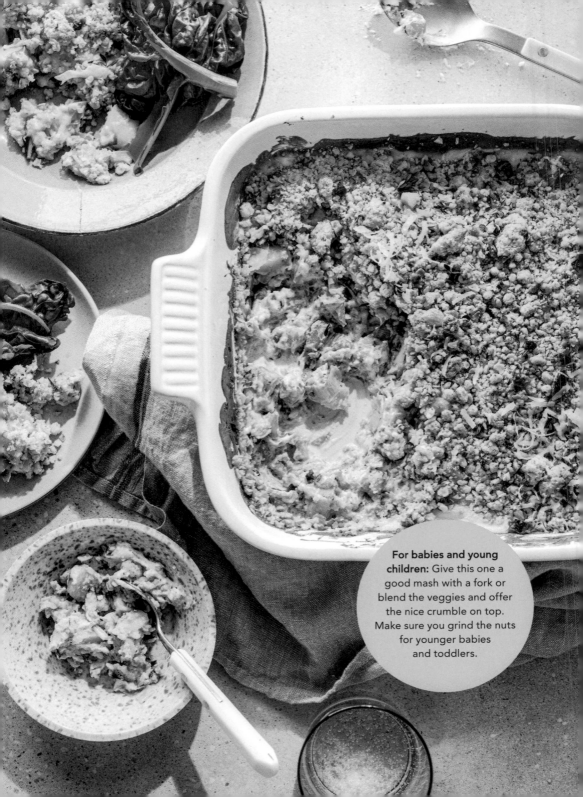

For babies and young children: Give this one a good mash with a fork or blend the veggies and offer the nice crumble on top. Make sure you grind the nuts for younger babies and toddlers.

CREAMY VEG CRUMBLE

I really wanted to include a savoury crumble recipe in this book, and was inspired to create this really delicious and hearty dinner dish. I've made this multiple times for family and friends and it's always a hit! It's a little longer in terms of prep, but makes a fairly big amount, so you can easily have leftovers the next day or freeze for when you need them.

Serves: Family of 4 plus plenty of leftovers
Prep time: 40 minutes
Cook time: 1 hour 10 minutes

1.25kg mixed veg (I used carrots, leek and parsnips), peeled and cut into 2–3cm chunks (keep them all roughly the same size)
drizzle of olive oil
175g plain flour
50g porridge oats
125g unsalted butter
50g ground or roughly chopped nuts (I use hazelnuts or walnuts – grind if offering to young babies)
50g cheddar cheese, grated
2 garlic cloves, crushed
¼ tsp ground nutmeg
600ml milk of choice
3 sprigs of thyme, leaves picked
steamed greens or green salad, to serve

1. Preheat the oven to 220°C/200°C fan. Spread the veg out over a baking tray, drizzle with the oil and toss to coat. Roast in the oven for 30 minutes, turning the veg halfway through, until lightly golden and tender.

2. Meanwhile, put 125g of the flour in a bowl with the porridge oats, then put this on the scales. Melt the butter in a medium saucepan, then pour 75g of it into the flour mixture.

3. Add the ground or chopped nuts and the grated cheese and stir until you have a sandy, slightly biscuity crumble mixture. Set aside.

4. To make the white sauce, put the remaining flour into the pan of the remaining melted butter and place over a medium-high heat. Cook, stirring, for 2–3 minutes, until the mixture has become drier and smells biscuity, then stir in the garlic and the nutmeg and cook for 2 minutes more. Gradually whisk in the milk, stirring constantly and keeping it over the heat – it will seize and thicken at first, then gradually thin out into a sauce that easily coats the back of a spoon. Stir in the thyme leaves and set aside.

5. Once the vegetables are cooked, transfer them to a large baking dish and pour over the white sauce. Stir gently to coat everything thoroughly, then scatter over the crumble, patting it down to pack it in slightly.

6. Bake for 40 minutes, until the crumble is light golden and the sauce is bubbling up around the edges. Allow to stand for 5 minutes, then serve with steamed greens or a green salad. To batch cook you can use two smaller pie dishes instead of one large one, and freeze one of them before baking.

CHEAT'S VEGGIE LASAGNE

I love a lasagne, but also find myself not cooking them often because they can take quite a long time. So, I wanted to create a lasagne recipe that was super easy. There is no pre-cooking of individual elements first, and no béchamel, which saves lots of time. If you can grate the vegetables in a food processor it's even quicker, as this is the only thing that takes a while. It's really tasty and has been such a hit with my whole family. You can swap the lasagne sheets for layers of pasta, and I've tried it with both fresh and dried lasagne and it works well. This recipe makes loads so you're bound to have leftovers!

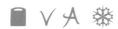

Serves: 4 with plenty of leftovers
Prep time: 20 minutes
Cook time: 30–40 minutes

1 garlic clove, crushed or finely grated
2 carrots, peeled and coarsely grated
1 or 2 sweet potatoes (about 300g), coarsely grated
2 x 400g tins chopped tomatoes
1 tbsp dried oregano
250g pre-cooked lentils e.g., puy or green lentils
600g cottage cheese or dairy-free alternative
150g grated mozzarella, plus 40g for sprinkling on top (or dairy-free alt)
200g packet of fresh lasagne sheets (dried work too, but might take a little longer to cook)
steamed greens or a simple salad, to serve

For babies and young children: Babies who are still experimenting with solid foods may need this to be lightly blended. Or you could roll up the lasagne sheets and give the sauce a blend. Older babies will probably be happy to play with and dissect this a little, and eat some with their hands and some off a spoon. Let them explore.

1. Preheat the oven to 200°C/180°C fan.
2. Grate the vegetables (garlic, carrots, sweet potato) into a large bowl. Squeeze out any excess liquid, by wrapping the grated veg in a paper towel and pressing firmly. Then add back into the bowl and tip in the tinned tomatoes, dried oregano and lentils. Give it a good mix and pop to one side.
3. In another bowl, mix the cottage cheese and 150g of the grated mozzarella.
4. Spoon a third of the tomato and lentil mix into an ovenproof dish or tin (about 20 x 30cm), then lay down the lasagne sheets. Top with 4 heaped tablespoons (about a third) of the cottage cheese mix, spreading it right to the sides, then add another third of the tomato and lentil mix, then more lasagne sheets and another third of the creamy mix. Finish with a third layer of lasagne sheets and the remaining creamy mix, and a little extra cheese for the top.
5. Bake in the oven for 30–40 minutes or until golden and bubbling. Serve with steamed greens or a simple salad.

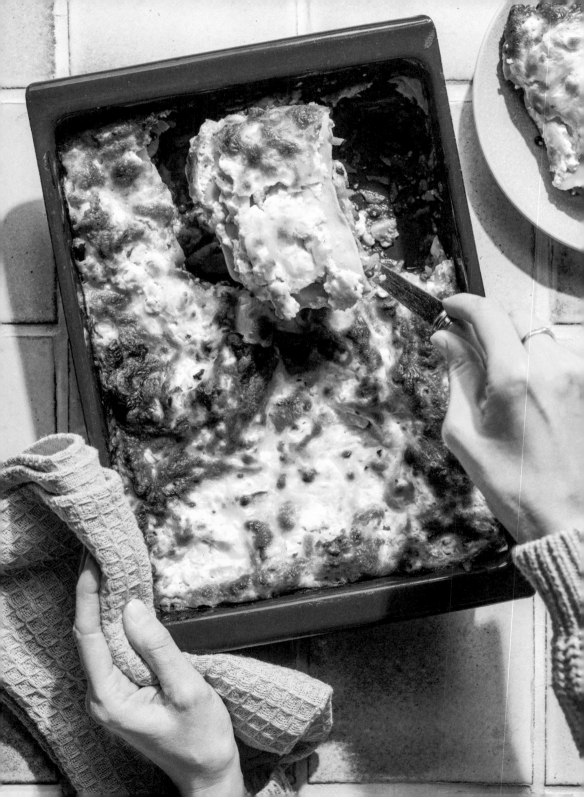

LEFTOVER VEG TRAYBAKE

At home we're huge fans of Mediterranean veggies, so we often have plenty of these in the fridge, and sometimes that means leftovers that we need to use up. That's why I came up with this traybake recipe – to help you use up all those veggies that you don't want to waste. Use whatever veggies you have, anything goes! There is a bit of an in-and-out-of-the-oven with this one, but it's a matter of chopping them up and bunging them into the tray.

Serves: 4, with leftovers
Prep time: 20 minutes
Cook time: 1 hour 10 minutes

1.2kg base veg (e.g. 1 red onion, 1 fennel,
    1 aubergine, 1 courgette, 1 pepper,
    2 carrots, or whatever you have leftover
    in the fridge), trimmed, deseeded where
    needed and cut into 2cm chunks
500g small potatoes, halved, or larger ones
    cut into 2cm chunks
oil, for drizzling
a few sprigs of fresh herbs such as rosemary
    or thyme (or 1 tbsp dried oregano)
300g fresh cherry tomatoes
2 garlic cloves, roughly chopped or crushed
400g tin chopped tomatoes
60g buffalo mozzarella (or feta)
    or dairy-free alternative, to serve
handful of pine nuts (optional – only
    for older children and adults)

1. Preheat the oven to 200°C/180°C fan. Pop all the prepped base veggies (onions, fennel, aubergine etc), plus the potatoes into a large roasting tray (approx 30cm x 35cm), or two if your trays aren't that big. Drizzle with a little oil and the herbs, and toss together.

2. Roast for 30 mins until looking lovely and golden. Then add the fresh tomatoes and garlic (divide between two if using two trays), cook for 10 minutes, then pour in the tinned tomatoes and a tin (400mls) of hot water, mix about and pop back into the oven for another 30 mins until thickened and flavours combined.

3. Serve topped with a little feta cheese crumbled on top or mozzarella torn over and a scattering of toasted pine nuts (optional).

For babies and young children: Leave off the pine nuts and make sure that the veggies are super soft for young babies and toddlers. You could always blend the veggies here into a sauce and offer some of the potatoes for them to dip in instead.

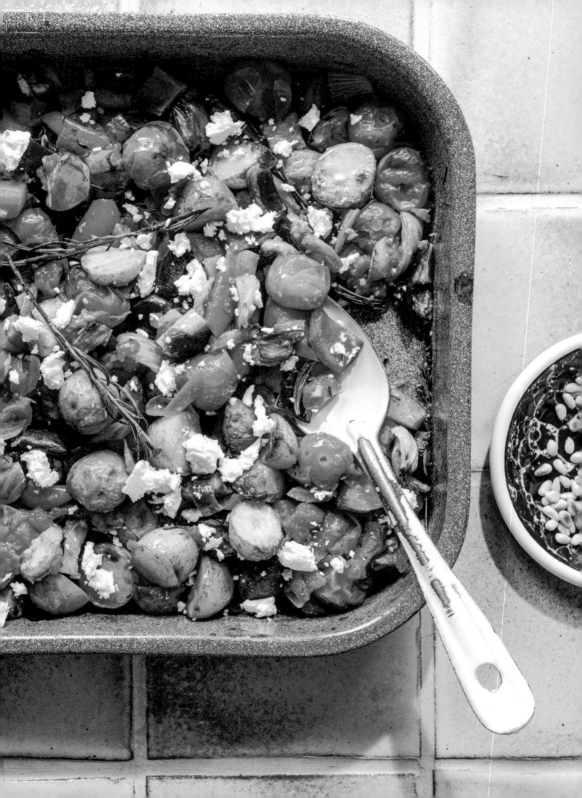

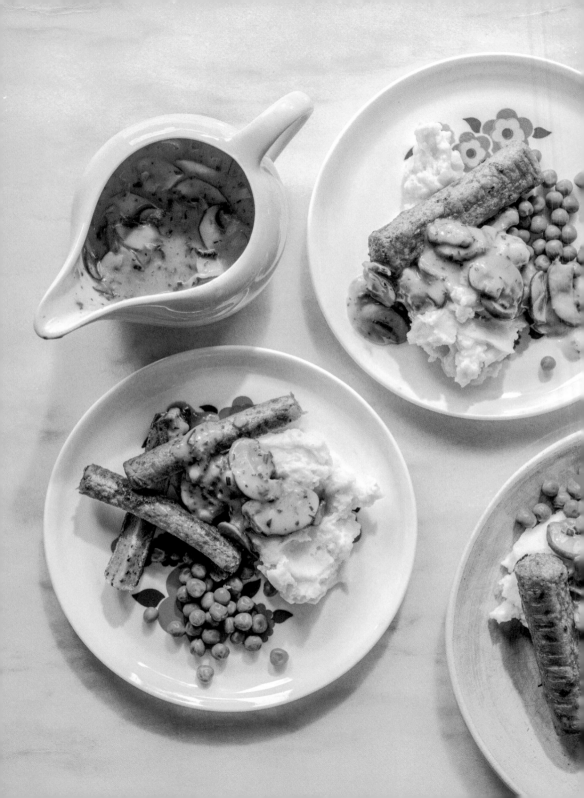

VEGGIE BANGERS & MASH WITH MUSHROOM GRAVY

Bangers and Mash is an absolute classic recipe that I just had to include in this book. This is my veggie take on it, with a few added extras and a couple of little twists (of course). You can make this with meat sausages just the same. It's so hearty and doesn't take much hands-on time, apart from the mushroom gravy, which is a gamechanger in our house!

Serves: 4
Prep time: 20 minutes
Cook time: 20 minutes

6–8 frozen vegetarian sausages
    (I used Linda McCartney)
25g unsalted butter or spread
200g chestnut mushrooms, finely sliced
3 rosemary sprigs, picked and finely chopped
2 tbsps plain flour
500mls water/low-salt stock
1 kilo maris piper potatoes, peeled and
    cut into 4cm chunks
a splash of milk

For babies and young children:
Try and choose lower salt sausages. Sausages do tend to be a little salty, so they aren't ideal for young babies.

If serving to slightly older children, make sure you slice them into quarters as they can be a choking hazard for children under 5.

1. Preheat the oven to 200°C/180°C fan. Put the sausages onto a lined baking tray and cook according to the packet instructions (usually 10–12 minutes), turning them halfway, until lovely and golden.
2. Meanwhile, bring a large pan of water to the boil, add the potatoes and cook for 12 minutes or so, until soft. Drain and leave to steam dry, then mash well, adding a splash of milk (and a little extra butter if you fancy!) until smooth and creamy.
3. Meanwhile, melt the butter or spread in a large frying pan – on a high heat, add the mushrooms and rosemary and cook for 5 minutes, stirring occasionally, until cooked and smelling delicious.
4. Turn to a medium heat then add the plain flour to the pan, and mix about to form a thick mixture. Slowly add the stock/water, turning the heat up slightly again and mixing each time before adding any more stock/water, to create your mushroom gravy. It will take around 10–15 minutes until thick and pourable.
5. Serve the gravy alongside the mash, sausages and some green veggies. Season to taste for adults, if needed.

Celebrations

BEETROOT, APPLE AND SWEET POTATO CRISPS

I love veggie crisps, and these ones are insanely good! There's a bit of in and out of the oven to get them nicely crisp and not burnt, so they aren't ones you'll do every day. But they are great to bring out at a party – making a different, exciting and colourful spread. Great for a party!

Serves: 4–6
Prep time: 10 minutes
Cook time: 15–30 minutes

1 medium beetroot
1 medium apple
1 medium sweet potato, peeled

1. Preheat the oven to 170°C/150°C fan. Line two large baking trays with baking paper.
2. You can prep the fruit or veg one of two ways to get them the same consistency of thin, crisp shavings: either with a mandoline (with a guard to protect your hands), or you can peel them with a speed peeler.
3. Lay the slices on the tray. Bake in the oven for 15–20 minutes. Then turn over and bake for a further 5–10 minutes until golden and crispy. Some of the fruit and veg might need a little longer depending on how thin they are, so keep checking so they don't burn!
4. Remove from the oven and leave the crisps to cool a little, then carefully remove from the trays. Serve some immediately, and pop the rest in an airtight container. They will keep well for a few days.

EASY PEACHY SPONGE

When my parents made this the kids went wild, so I wanted to share it with you all. You can change the tinned fruit you use, depending on what you have in the cupboard – it is super quick and delicious.

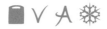

Serves: 4, plus leftovers
Prep time: 5 minutes
Cook time: 25–30 minutes

2 free-range eggs or 2 flaxseed eggs (see page 108)
140g butter, softened (at room temperature) or spread, plus extra for greasing
45g caster sugar
170g self-raising flour
2 x 227g tins peach slices in juice syrup, roughly chopped (reserving the syrup)
natural yoghurt or Sugar-free Banana Custard (page 195), to serve

1. Preheat the oven to 200°C/180°C fan and grease an ovenproof baking dish (about 20 x 20cm) with a little butter or spread.
2. Mix the butter (or spread) and sugar in a bowl, then add the eggs/flaxseed eggs, flour and reserved peach syrup and mix to combine.
3. Put the peaches on the bottom of the baking dish then pour over the sponge mix. Smooth it out evenly and bake in the middle of the oven for 25–30 minutes, or until cooked through and golden.
4. Remove from the oven and serve warm. Serve with some natural yoghurt or banana custard drizzled over.

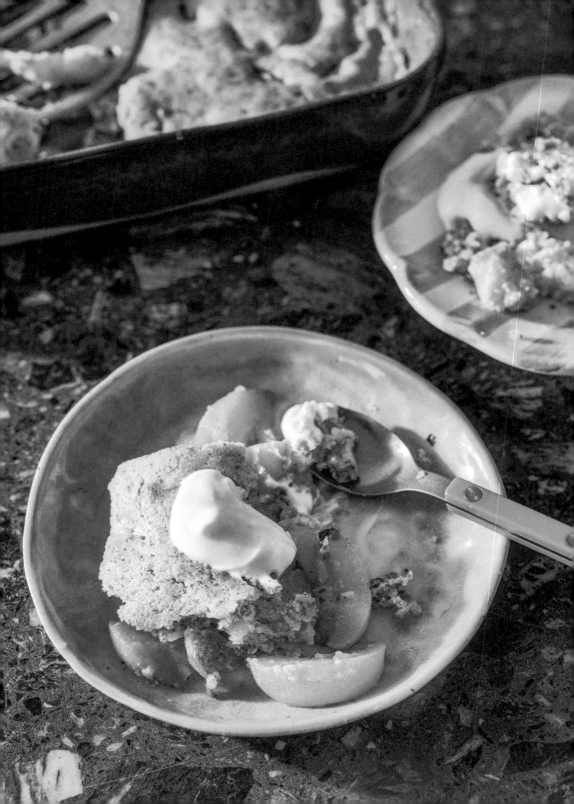

LOWER-SUGAR MARBLE CAKE

This is such a simple cake and, like most of my Celebrations recipes, it's much lower in sugar than your average. I love this cake – it reminds me of being on holiday and having cake for breakfast! It's super light and fluffy, and even though it's lower in sugar it's still nice and sweet. You can make it into a classic marble loaf cake if you like – which is the more traditional shape – but I wanted to make this into a recipe you could turn into a perfect birthday cake for the whole family; it is a great party piece, make double the batter to turn it into a layered cake. It is perfect for getting the kids involved too.

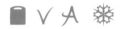

Makes: a single layer cake (double up the recipe to make another layer)
Prep time: 10 minutes
Cook time: 25–30 minutes

80g Greek yoghurt
4 tbsp olive oil
90g light brown sugar
80ml milk of choice
1 large free-range egg or
    1 flaxseed egg (see page 108)
150g plain flour
2 tsp baking powder
1½ tbsp cocoa powder

FOR THE TOPPING
100g Greek yoghurt
1 tbsps of icing sugar,
150g fresh strawberries and/or
    raspberries, trimmed.

Cook's tip: If you are doubling the mixture and making a layered cake, you could fill it with chia seed jam (see page 203) and natural yoghurt.

1. Preheat the oven to 200°C/180°C fan. Grease a loose-bottomed 20cm cake tin. If using a flaxseed egg, make this now.
2. In a large bowl (or stand mixer) whisk the yoghurt, oil and sugar until combined. Stir in the milk and egg (or flaxseed egg), then mix in the flour and baking powder.
3. Pour half the cake mix into the tin, then mix the cocoa powder in the remaining mix in the bowl to create chocolate batter. Pour into the cake tin and swirl through the plain vanilla mix. Smooth out the top and bake for 25–30 minutes or until it is cooked through and golden on top.
4. Remove from the oven. Let the cake cool in the tin for 5 minutes then carefully remove from the tin and allow to cool completely on a rack.
5. Once the cake has cooled completely, sprinkle it with some icing sugar, and top with some strawberries/raspberries. If you are making a double layer then spread a little chia seed jam (page 203) and a good dollop of thick natural Greek yoghurt onto the cake, then place the other marble cake on top and dust with icing sugar.

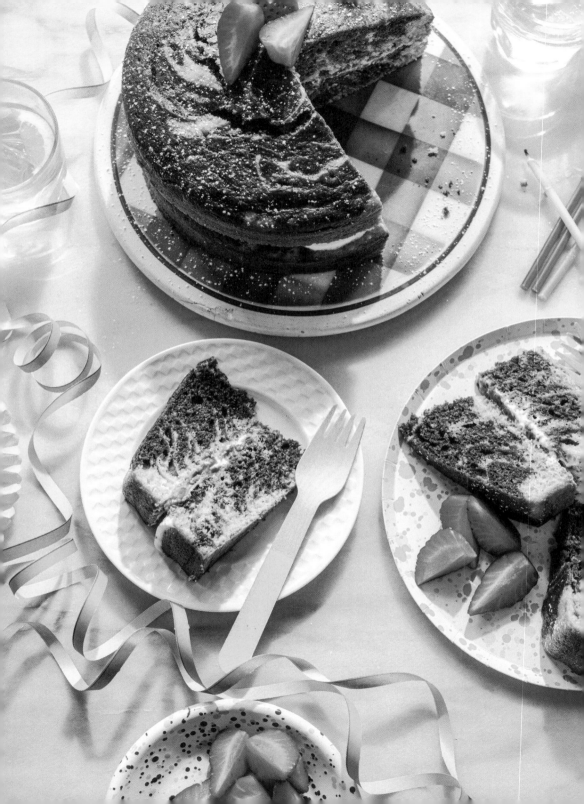

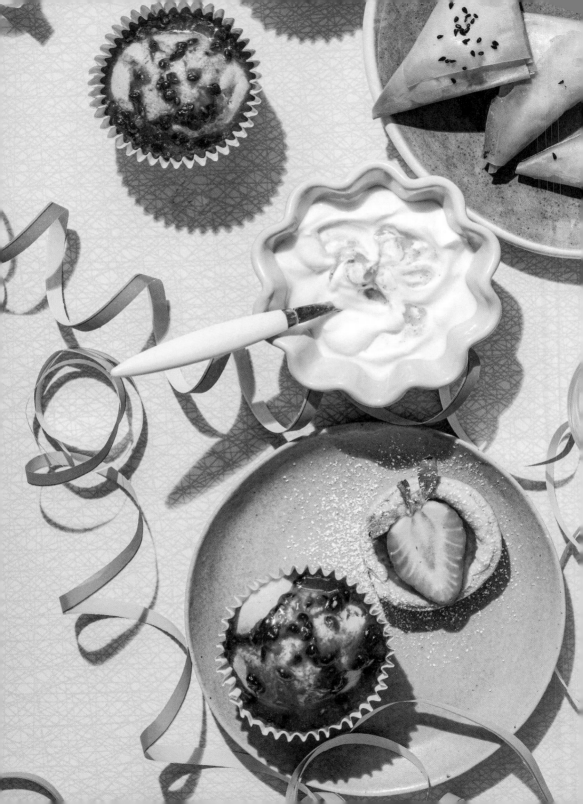

FAIRY CAKES

In this book I wanted to include family-friendly bakes that do contain sugar, but a lower amount than you get in typical recipes. I always think about ways to make recipes a bit different, and often find that it's easy to simply reduce the sugar in cakes, while still ensuring they taste delicious. So here are my lower-sugar fairy cakes, perfect for any occasion and easy to make!

 V

Makes: 10–12 fairy cakes
Prep time: 10–15 minutes
Cook time: 15–20 minutes

150g unsalted butter or spread
90g caster sugar
3 large free-range eggs
3 tsp vanilla extract
240g self-raising flour
4 tbsp milk of choice

FOR THE ICING (OPTIONAL)
50g soft fruit such as strawberries, raspberries or blackberries, washed and mashed
50–60g icing sugar

1. Preheat the oven to 200°C/180°C fan.
2. Pop cupcake cases into a 12-hole cupcake/muffin tin.
3. Mix the butter and sugar in a bowl (of a food processor, or stand mixer). Then add the eggs and vanilla and mix again. Sift in the self-raising flour and combine.
4. Add the milk a little at at time until you get a slightly thinner texture that you can easily dollop into cupcake cases.
5. Divide the mix between the 12 cases and bake in the middle of the oven for 15–20 minutes until golden and cooked through. Leave to cool for 5 minutes, then remove to a cooling rack.
6. Meanwhile, if you are using, make some icing – add the mashed fruit to the icing sugar and mix until combined. Drizzle over the cooled cupcakes. Or, just sprinkle over some icing sugar, and pop a little mashed fruit on top for smaller babies.

For young children: Mash a little fruit with the back of a fork and add to the top instead of the icing sugar. It's best to avoid offering this until they are a little older and more 'aware' of cakes.

BEETROOT BROWNIE

I love this brownie so much: it's utterly delicious and a really special recipe. It does contain some added sugar, but it's much less than you'd normally find in a brownie; and it also has beetroot for some extra nutrients. The taste of the earthy beetroot works so well with the chocolate and it's a winner all round for my family.

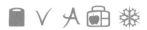

Makes: 16 brownies
Prep time: 10 minutes
Cook time: 20–25 minutes

250g vacuum-packed cooked beetroot in natural juices (not vinegar!)
150g good quality dark chocolate (minimum 70% cocoa solids), roughly chopped
80g unsalted butter or spread, cold, plus extra for greasing
3 large free-range eggs, beaten or 3 flaxseed eggs (see page 108)
150g caster sugar
100g self-raising flour
1 heaped tbsp cocoa powder

1. Preheat the oven to 190°C/170°C fan. Grease and line a 20cm square brownie tin with greaseproof paper.
2. Drain the beetroot and leave it in a sieve.
3. Melt the dark chocolate – either pop it in the microwave for 2–3 minutes, stirring every 30 seconds until all melted, or place in a heatproof bowl on top of a small saucepan of simmering water and let it gently melt.
4. Whizz up the beetroot, butter and melted chocolate in a food processor until smooth, then pour into a large bowl.
5. Add the eggs or flaxseed eggs and sugar and mix again, then mix in the flour and cocoa until combined.
6. Pour into the greased and lined brownie tin and bake in the oven for 20–25 minutes until cooked through but still with a little wobble (this will make sure you have a little gooey centre).
7. Leave to cool completely in the tin, then cut into 16 squares.

For babies and young children: It's best to avoid offering this until babies and young children are a little older and more 'aware' of cakes and chocolates.

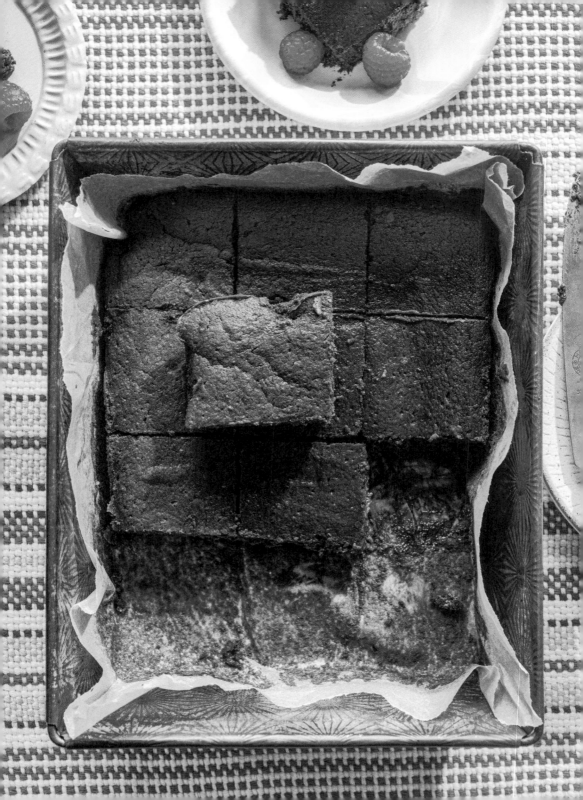

APPLE AND FOREST FRUIT MARZIPAN CRUMBLE

This makes a double batch of crumble topping, so you will have extra in the freezer ready for another time to top another one – winner! Although the marzipan is in the title, this is optional as I know that marzipan can be really divisive. You can easily leave it out if you prefer, but it does add a bit of je ne sais quoi to this recipe.

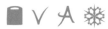

Serves: 4, with leftovers
Makes: extra 720g crumble topping
Prep time: 15 minutes
Cook time: 30–35 minutes

2 large eating apples (approx 350g)
250g frozen forest fruits like blueberries, blackberries & raspberries
1 orange, juiced or 40mls apple/orange juice
150g unsalted butter, cold and cubed, or dairy-free alt
150g wholemeal plain flour
1 tsp of ground cinnamon
50g golden caster sugar (optional – leave out for babies and toddlers)
200g oats
50g milled seeds (e.g. pumpkin, sunflower)
100g marzipan, coarsely grated (optional)

> **For babies and young children:** Leave out the marzipan and the sugar.

1. Preheat the oven to 200°C/180°C fan. Peel the apples and coarsely grate (leaving the core). Add to a 20 x 25cm ovenproof dish with the frozen fruit, juice of the orange juice (or apple/orange juice) and mix to make your filling.
2. Add the butter, flour and cinnamon to a large bowl.
3. Pulse with a hand blender until you have a breadcrumb texture. Or, if using your hands, rub between your thumb and finger to create little crumbs.
4. Stir in the sugar (if using), oats and seeds, and mix altogether. Now is the time to add the grated marzipan, if using. Stir to mix with the topping.
5. Now divide the topping into two, and put one batch into a bag in the freezer for another time. Sprinkle the other half on top of the fruit.
6. Bake in the middle of the oven for 30 minutes, or until golden and smelling delicious. Leave to cool slightly before serving with a dollop of natural yoghurt, or no-sugar custard.

SUGAR-FREE BANANA CUSTARD

My kids love custard, so I wanted to create a recipe which was simple and delicious but didn't have all the added sugar. This can be served alone, topped with fruit, or on top of this crumble, and also works really well with the Easy Peachy Sponge on page 186.

Makes: 400ml
Prep time: 5 minutes
Cook time: 8–10 minutes

360ml milk of choice
2 medium ripe bananas, peeled
1 tbsp cornflour
2 large free-range eggs or
    2 flaxseed eggs (see page 108)
1 tsp vanilla essence (optional)

1. Put the milk and bananas into a blender jug and blend on high until combined and lump-free.
2. Add the cornflour and eggs and blend again until combined, then pour into a medium saucepan and add the vanilla (if using). Cook over a medium heat for 3–5 minutes, stirring continuously, or until thickened and smooth.

Cook's tip: If using flaxseed egg, bear in mind that it will have a slightly different colour, and won't be as thick as if made with eggs.

If the cooked custard seems a little thick and lumpy/grainy, blend it up quickly to get rid of the lumps!

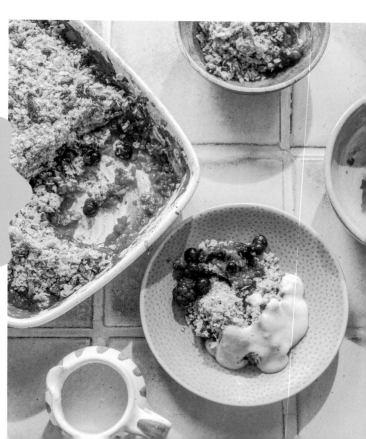

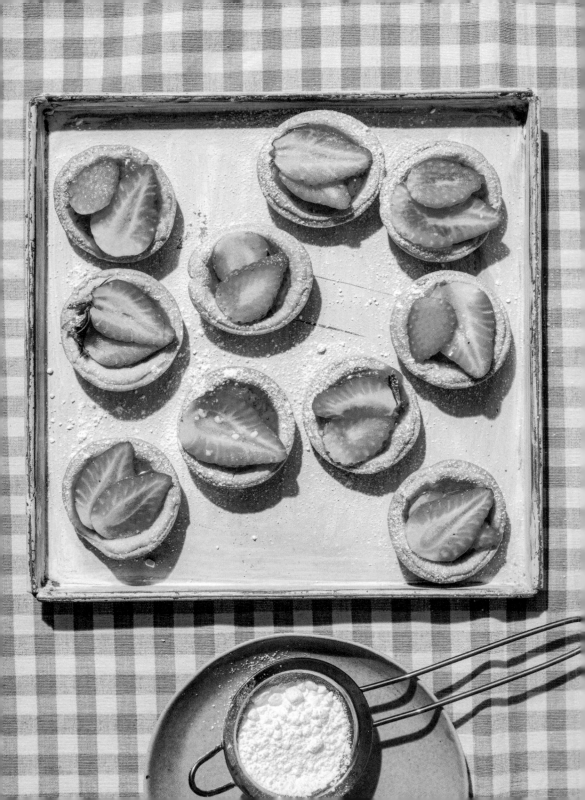

STRAWBERRY TARTS

I had the idea for these when my mum came round with some pastry cases and a punnet of strawberries. We bunged it together and Ada went wild for them! I added a little extra with the coulis and voila, a new snack was born. We love these, so simple and so delicious and they look great too!

Makes: 12 tarts
Prep time: 10 minutes (if you have made pastry already)
Cook time: 15–20 minutes

2 x 230g punnet of strawberries
icing sugar, to taste (optional)
All-Purpose Quick Pastry (see page 218) or shop-bought pastry

For babies and young children: Once they are au fait with finger foods these can be a great one for babies to explore and self-feed. Leave out the icing for babies and toddlers.

1. Preheat the oven to 200°C/180°C fan.
2. Roll out the pastry to 1–2 mm thick, cut out 12 x 7–8 cm rounds (a small glass will do). You might need to re-roll the pastry. Lay each round into a shallow cupcake tray, pushing the pastry circle into the hole. Bake for 10–12 minutes, until golden and cooked.
3. While the pastry is baking, trim 360g of the strawberries, and cut into small pieces. Put into a medium saucepan with a splash of water (you can add a teaspoon of icing sugar to add a little sweetness, if you like).
4. Cook on high-medium heat for 5–6 minutes, stirring occasionally and mashing it down a little to create a coulis. Decant into a bowl and leave to one side to cool.
5. Meanwhile, trim and finely slice the remaining strawberries.
6. Once the pastry is baked, divide the coulis between the bases, then top with the cut strawberries.
7. Sprinkle with icing sugar, if using, and serve.

2-INGREDIENT SORBET

Everyone loves ice cream, and this sorbet is creamy, easy to make, super delicious and has no added sugar. Great for summer BBQs and parties, or just a delicious ice-cold hit of sweetness. Once you've made it, you'll always want to have some in your freezer!

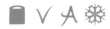

Serves: 6
Prep time: 10 minutes
Freeze time: 2 hours

150g natural yoghurt or dairy-free alternative
350g frozen fruit/smoothie/tropical
    fruit mix (e.g. banana/raspberry/
    strawberry/mango mix)

FOR TOPPING (OPTIONAL)
coconut shavings
dark chocolate, grated
finely ground nuts

1. In a food processor, add the frozen fruit and blend until all the fruit is broken up and mixed.
2. Add the yoghurt and blend again until combined. Serve immediately (or follow on below and serve another day/later).
3. If serving later, decant into a freezer container with a lid.
4. Leave in the freezer for at least 2 hours, then take it out for 5–10 minutes before serving to soften slightly (enough to scoop).
5. Scoop into bowls and top with some coconut shavings, dark chocolate or finely blended nuts, if you like.

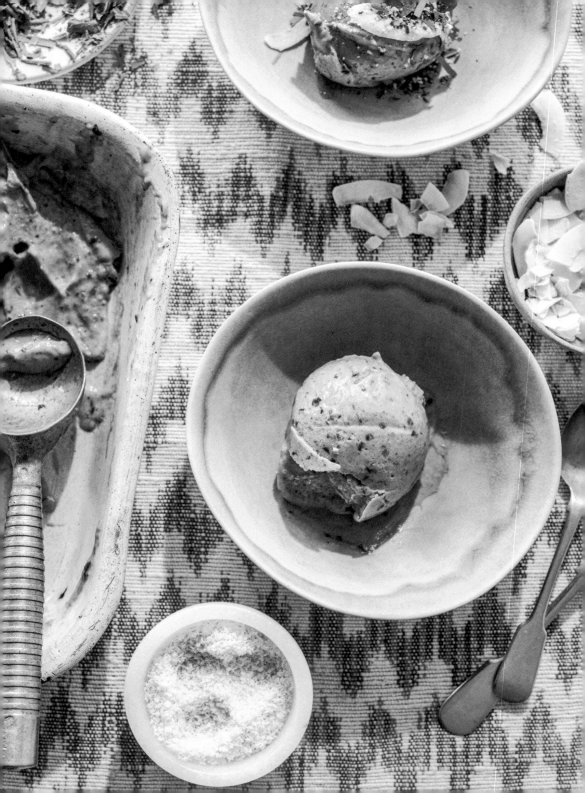

Snacks, Sides and Bakes

SIMPLE CHEESY CRACKERS

 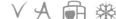

Lovely little crackers to bring out at a party or to have as part of a snack. They also go so well with the Mexican soup recipe on page 160 as a little cheesy side. These have lower levels of salt than shop-bought crackers or crisps, and I've tried to add some extra nutrients in.

Makes: 18–20 crackers
Prep time: 10 minutes
Cook time: 12–15 minutes

50g almond flour (if you don't have this, just use 50g additional self-raising flour)
100g self-raising flour
80g unsalted butter, cubed, room temp
50g cheese, grated
½ tbsp of small seeds e.g. flaxseeds, sunflower seeds

1. Preheat oven to 200°C/180°C fan.
2. Mix the flours and the butter together in a bowl and combine with your hands until it forms breadcrumbs.
3. Add the cheese and seeds and mix it all together between your fingers and hands, until it rolls easily into a ball.
4. Roll the ball out onto a floured surface until it's around 0.5cm thick and use a stamper to cut out shapes. Re-roll and keep stamping until you've used all the dough.
5. Lay them on a greaseproof covered baking tray and bake in the oven for 12–15 mins.
6. Once out, let them firm up and cool down for 5 minutes on a cooling rack before serving!

For babies and young children: These are nice and crumbly and don't contain extra salt, so are fine to offer as little finger foods.

CARROT, DATE AND COCONUT ENERGY BALLS

I love carrots, they give a great sweetness while providing some nutrients. This is a super quick recipe (and you can mix it up with other things if you don't have all of it in). This is a fab one to bring out for picnics and play dates, and easy to freeze and store too.

Makes: 16–18 balls
Prep time: 5 minutes, plus 30 minutes chilling

1 medium carrot (about 65g), peeled and coarsely grated
8 medjool dates (about 160g), stones removed
100g unsalted nuts (almonds, brazil nuts)
2–3 tbsp desiccated coconut (optional)

1. Put the carrot, dates and nuts in a food processor and blitz until combined.
2. Transfer the mixture to a bowl then take tablespoons of the mix and roll them into 16–18 balls (about the size of a golf ball). Roll some in desiccated coconut if you fancy.
3. Pop the balls onto a lined tray and put in the fridge for about 30 minutes to set a little, then dig in.
4. Store in the fridge in a sealed container for up to 2–3 weeks.

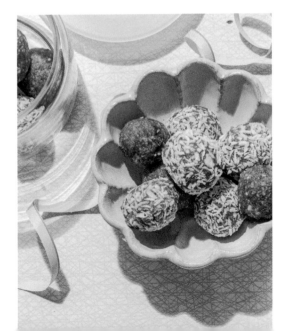

BLACKBERRY CHIA SEED JAM

Prep time: 5 minutes
Cook time: 10–15 minutes

A super simple and delicious jam recipe. Blackberries can be a little tart, so the sugar helps to offset it. My two love jam, so this one is a winner. You can easily make it without the sugar.

250g frozen blackberries
a few splashes of water
4 tsp chia seeds
1 tbsp sugar (or jam sugar) (optional)

1. Add blackberries and water to a pan on a medium to high heat, and allow the blackberries to defrost. Once defrosted, give them a good mash and add the chia seeds and sugar (if using) and stir through.
2. Allow the mixture to bubble for around 5 mins and then give it another stir and a mash down and allow it to cook for another few minutes. Then let it sit for 5 mins.

PANGRATTATO TOPPING

This crunchy little topping is something I use to add texture and nutrients to many dishes like traybakes, soups and pastas – it's especially good with the Cheesy Greens Pasta on page 140.

35g whole almonds
50g stale bread
1 sprig of thyme, leaves picked
½ garlic clove, peeled and chopped

1. Whizz up the ingredients in a high-speed blender until finely ground.
2. Fry in a frying pan on medium heat with a little oil, until golden and crisp.
3. Allow to cool and serve immediately, or store in a sealed container in the fridge for up to 2 weeks.

For babies and young children: It's so easy to leave out the sugar on this one, the jam will be a little tart, but it's great to expose them to a range of tastes and flavours.

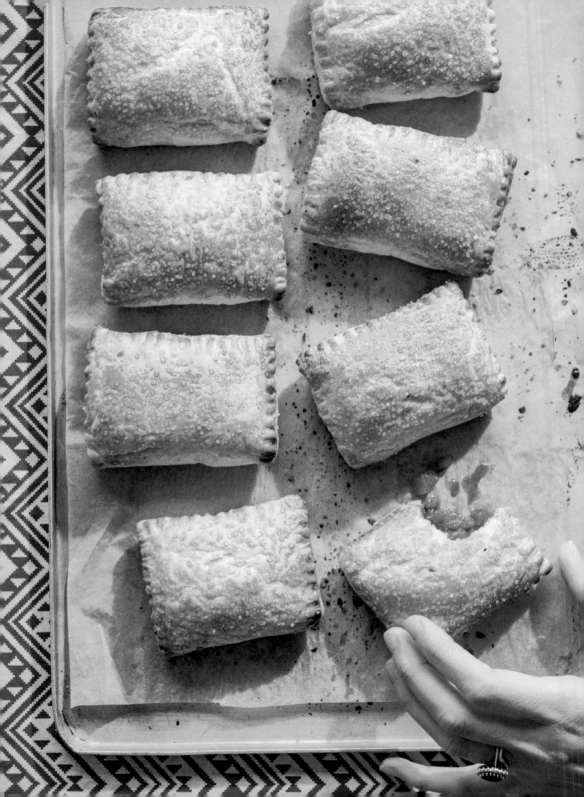

ON-THE-GO APPLE AND BLACKBERRY PARCEL

This has been an absolute hit in our house. Super easy to make and tastes amazing. Definitely one you'll struggle not to gobble up before the kids get home from school. This is a staple in my freezer, and one that I use as snacks, for breakfast or as a 'pudding'! A total winner. Remember that on coming out of the oven the insides will be piping hot, so do let them cool a lot before serving.

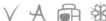

Makes: 8 parcels
Prep time: 15 minutes
Cook time: 25–35 minutes

2 medium apples, approx 350g peeled and cored, cut into small ½ cm chunks
a handful (approx) 40g frozen blackberries
160mls of apple juice
320g sheet of pre-rolled puff pastry
milk of choice for glazing
a little Demerara sugar (optional, to top)

For babies and young children:
Make sure you leave it to cool down before eating! The insides get so hot, you don't want kids to burn their mouths. Cut into little sticks for babies and leave off the sugar.

1. Preheat the oven to 210°C/190°C fan.
2. Put the apples and blackberries into a medium saucepan with the apple juice, and cook on a medium-high heat for 10–15 minutes, until the apples are cooked and the blackberries are broken down.
3. Roughly mash up with the spoon to create a chunky apple and blackberry compote. Leave to cool completely.
4. Lay the pastry out on a floured surface and cut into half lengthways, then cut into four lengths horizontally. So you end up with 8 rectangular pieces of pastry.
5. Divide the mix equally and place at the end of each piece of pastry, leaving 1cm at the edge, reserving any spare apple/blackberry juice for glazing with the milk. Fold over the end to reach the other side then seal it with a fork making a pretty edge on 3 sides.
6. Pop on a lined baking tray, brush with some milk and some of the leftover mashed up fruit. Sprinkle with a little sugar if you fancy and then bake for 15–20 minutes, until golden and crispy.

FRUITY CHEESECAKE BARK

I always love the look of these fruity barks, and this one really is beautiful – a great centrepiece for dessert, and wonderful in the summertime too. A super simple and fun recipe. Get the kids to help out, and go mad on the sprinkling!

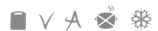

Makes: One sheet of bark
Prep time: 5 minutes
Freeze time: 1–2 hours

100g fresh strawberries, washed and hulled
450g thick Greek yoghurt
    (or dairy-free alternative)
150g cream cheese (or dairy-free alternative)
2 tsp vanilla essence
15g freeze-dried fruit (e.g., strawberries,
    raspberries, apple), crushed or broken up
20g unsalted pistachios, finely chopped,
    ground for babies

1. Blend or mash up the strawberries. Line a large baking sheet with greaseproof paper and pop to one side.
2. Mix the yoghurt, cream cheese and vanilla in a bowl until smooth. Swirl the mixture through the mashed-up strawberries then spread it out onto the lined tray, then scatter over the fruit and nuts.
3. Place in the freezer for 1–2 hours (or as long as you have!) until frozen, then break up into shards and serve immediately (it will quickly start to defrost). Or you can break off little bits to eat now, and save the rest in the freezer for another time!

For babies and young children: Grind or leave out the pistachios, and let it defrost a little before offering – it might get a little messy!

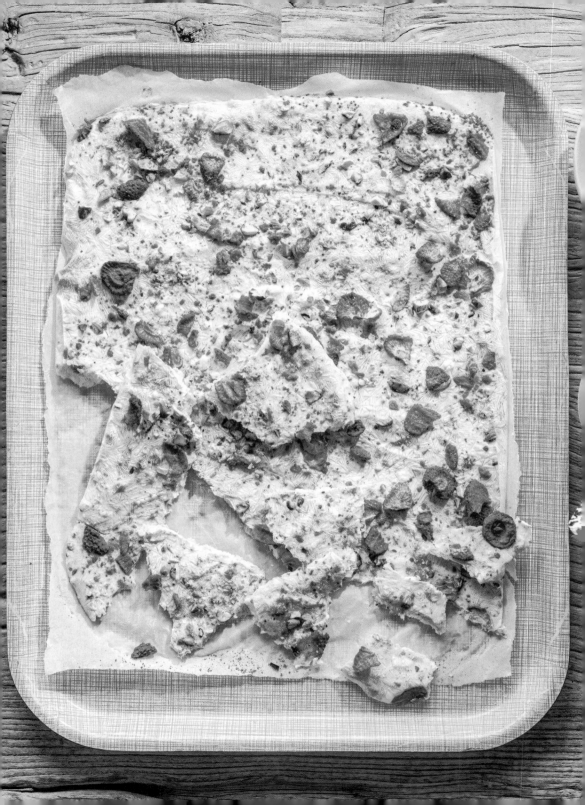

CHEESY PIZZA MUFFINS

This is a pizza-flavoured muffin – what's not to love? I totally love these pizza muffins – they are yummy, very moreish, and also easy to adapt and make vegan. Great for an on-the-go snack, lunchbox or even for brekkie, my freezer always has a stash! A great one to batch cook and freeze. Defrost the night before using.

 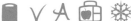

Makes: 12 muffins
Prep time: 10 minutes
Cook time: 15–20 minutes

165g tinned (drained) or frozen (defrosted) sweetcorn
1 garlic clove, chopped/crushed
50g butter or dairy-free spread, melted
10 cherry tomatoes, well chopped
2 tbsp tomato purée
½ bunch of basil (about 20g), finely chopped, or 1 tbsp dried oregano
2 large free-range eggs or 2 flaxseed eggs (see page 108)
60g grated mozzarella (or cheddar cheese, or dairy-free alternative), plus 20g extra for the top
100ml milk of choice
150g self-raising flour

1. Preheat the oven to 210°C/190°C fan. Line a 12-hole muffin tray with cupcake or muffin cases.
2. Put the sweetcorn in a large bowl along with the garlic, melted butter, tomatoes, tomato purée, basil, eggs (or flaxseed egg) and 60g of the cheese, give it a good mix then add the flour to make a thick batter.
3. Divide the mix evenly among the muffin cases and top with the remaining 20g of cheese.
4. Bake in the oven for 15–20 minutes or until cooked through, then remove from the oven and leave to cool a little before transferring to a cooling rack. Enjoy warm, or leave to cool completely and then eat, or pop them in the freezer for another day!

Cook's tip: To quickly defrost sweetcorn, run it under hot water in a colander

For babies and young children: Muffins usually work really well for babies as great little self-feeding options. If your baby is still figuring out finger foods you might want to cut them up into little sticks for them to hold and leave out the sweetcorn or give it a little blend first.

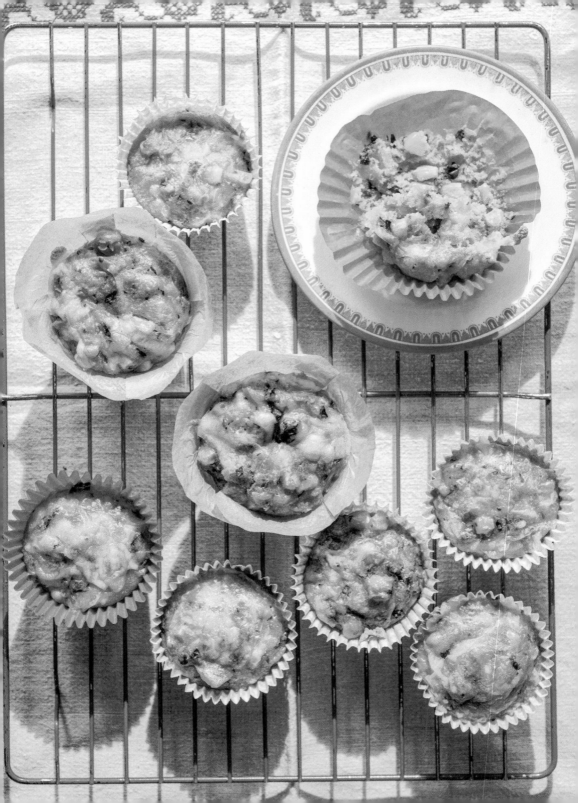

FROZEN VEG SCONES

My two love scones. It's always something that my mum brings round. Scones are a great family recipe, as a snack, with some soup or a salad. So I've tried to make an easy, cheap and wholesome scone recipe which should suit all!

Makes: 8–10 scones
Prep time: 15 minutes
Cook time: 10–15 minutes

200g frozen veg medley (such as sweetcorn, peas and carrots)
215g thick Greek yoghurt
100–120g red Leicester (or cheddar) cheese, coarsely grated
250g wholemeal self-raising flour, plus extra for dusting
1 tsp baking powder

1. Pop the frozen veg in a colander and pour over boiling water to defrost a little. Dab dry then leave to one side. Line 1 large baking tray with greaseproof paper. Preheat the oven to 200°C/180°C fan.
2. Mix the yoghurt and the frozen veg into a bowl then give it a good mix – keep mixing, it will come together. Then add 80g of the cheese, and the flour and mix it together. Use your hands to form the mixture into a ball, then pop it onto a floured surface, adding a little more flour if sticky to work with. Knead the dough for a few minutes until a little smoother.
3. Roll the dough out to an inch-thick piece. Using 7-cm cutters, cut out 8–10 scones. You can use the off cuts to re-roll until you can't make any more.
4. Drizzle with a little oil then sprinkle the rest of the cheese on top of each scone and bake in a lined tray for 20–25 minutes, or until cooked through.
5. Serve warm or leave to cool and serve.

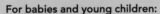

For babies and young children:
Once your baby is confident with self-feeding these will be a great option as the veg inside is nice and soft. Cut them into little scone sticks if you prefer. You might need to check any frozen veggies are not too hard.

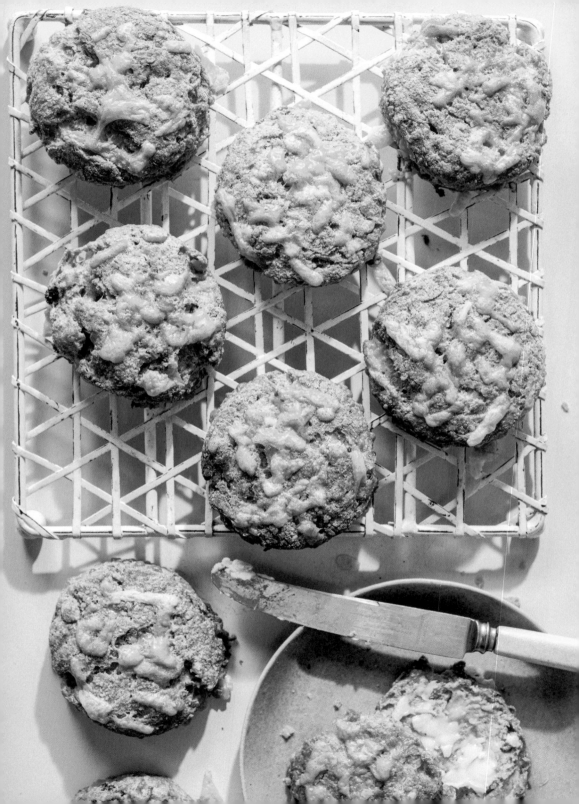

OATY COOKIE

A lovely little recipe and a warming, crumbly oaty biscuit which is super simple to make, and one that the kids will love to eat (and cook) too. Change it up with some chocolate chips if you'd like. This is a really simple and delicious recipe.

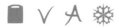

Makes: 10 cookies
Prep time: 10 minutes
Cook time: 10–12 minutes

125g oats
80g butter or spread
1 tbsp chia seeds, ground in a nutribullet
1 tbsp milk of choice
50g raisins or chocolate chips
1 tsp cinnamon
1 tbsp dark muscovado
1 tbsp peanut butter

1. Add the oats, butter, raisins, cinnamon, muscovado, peanut butter, ground chia seeds and milk to a bowl. Give it a good mix – it will come together, just keep mixing!
2. Roll into 10 balls the size of golf balls, pop onto a lined tray then squash down to flatten to disc shapes, approx 6cm-wide.
3. Bake for 10–12 minutes (or until golden) and cooked through. Transfer to a cooling rack and leave to cool and firm up a little.

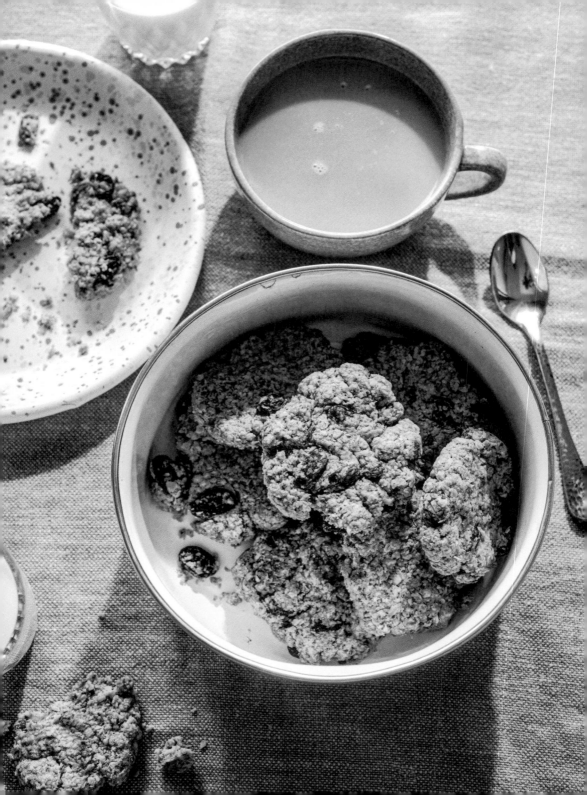

CAULIFLOWER CHEESE AND BUTTER BEAN MASH

I wanted to create a mash recipe that adds a little extra, and this cauliflower cheese, butter bean mash does just that. Added veggies, texture and flavours really changes up your standard mash – a great way to bring some variety if your kids love mashed potato!

 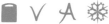

Serves: 4–6
Prep time: 5 minutes
Cook time: 15 minutes

500g potatoes, peeled
    & cut into 3–4cm chunks
350g fresh (or frozen) cauliflower,
    trimmed and cut into small
    chunks (stalk and all!)
a splash of milk, your choice
1 x 400g tin of butter beans, drained
50g mature cheddar cheese or red
    Leicester (or dairy-free alternative)

1. Fill a large saucepan with water and bring to the boil while prepping the rest of the vegetables. Add in the potatoes and cook for 15 minutes, adding the cauliflower halfway through, and the butterbeans a couple of minutes from the end, to heat through.
2. Drain the pan and leave for a few minutes to let the water evaporate and for the creamiest mash!
3. Mash the cauliflower, potatoes and butterbeans together until smooth, adding a splash of milk if needed. You might need to give it a really good mash together to get it nice and smooth.
4. Grate in the cheese, then mix again. Season with black pepper if you wish.

For babies and young children: Make sure the mash is nice and soft for young babies and there aren't any harder lumps throughout.

PESTO 3 WAYS

My family love pesto, and when you figure out how easy it can be to make, you might find this homemade pesto becomes a real staple in your household. This is a recipe you can do in three ways: the basic recipe, then freestyle with adding vegetables such as beetroot, red pepper or leftover greens. You may need a little extra nuts, as some ingredients are wetter than others. I'm sure you'll find these colourful pestos a winner!

Makes: approx 450g
Prep time: 5 minutes

BASIC RECIPE:
25g herb of choice, I like to use basil, parsley, coriander
a good squeeze of lemon
5 tbsp good-quality extra virgin olive oil
200g nuts, e.g. almonds, walnuts, pinenuts, pistachios
50g Parmesan (optional if keeping vegan!)

THEN ADD ONE FLAVOUR (USE 1, 2 OR 3)
1. 200g vacuum-pack beetroot, plus 1 tbsp of beetroot juice drained, OR
2. 150g roasted jarred red peppers, drained, OR
3. 100g leftover greens, like spinach, broccoli, kale, cavolo nero, peas – preferably cooked (will blend up better).

1. Pop all the ingredients into a food processor.
2. Whizz until combined – keep it chunkier if you like, or smoother depending on what you prefer. Add a splash of water if need be, to loosen a little.
3. Taste, and add a little more lemon/ Parmesan if needed.

VEGGIE SAMOSAS

These are great as a snack or part of lunch or a picnic, and also work brilliantly in lunch boxes. These can be a little fiddly, but it's worth it! I really like samosas, and haven't made my own many times before so this recipe was new and exciting. Definitely a nice one to make with slightly older kids.

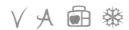

Makes: 12 samosas
Prep time: 15 minutes
Cook time: 35–40 minutes

sunflower oil for brushing
180g (1 large potato) potatoes, peeled and finely chopped
1 small onion, peeled and finely chopped or 5 spring onions
1 small carrot, peeled and coarsely grated
1 clove of garlic, peeled and finely chopped
½ tsp ground coriander
½ tsp ground cumin
½ tsp turmeric
50g of sultanas or raisins
60g frozen peas
3–4 large sheets of filo pastry (30x35cm sheets)
Greek yoghurt and mango chutney (optional, to serve)

1. Preheat the oven to 220°C/200°C fan. Line a baking tray with baking paper.
2. Heat a tablespoon of oil in a large frying pan over a medium heat. Add the onion/spring onions, garlic and carrot. Cook for 4–5 mins, stirring occasionally until soft and golden, adding the spices in for the final minute.
3. Stir to combine, then add the potatoes and 8–10 tablespoons of water so it covers the bottom of the pan, stirring to mix all the flavours together.
4. Turn the heat down to a low simmer and cover with a lid for 10–12 mins to cook the potatoes (until tender but still holding their shape).

5. Turn off the heat and add the peas and sultanas giving it all a good mix. Transfer the mix to a bowl and let it cool a little – 5 minutes will do – before filling.
6. Now to assemble the samosas: lay a sheet of filo on a clean surface. Cut into 7cm-wide strips.
7. Cover the rest of the filo with a damp cloth (to stop it drying out while you fill and fold).
8. Brush the strip with a little oil, then add a heaped tablespoon of filling, slightly to one side, in the top-right middle of one end of the strip.
9. Fold the top-left piece across into a triangle, keeping the filling in this shape. Then fold down into another triangle. Keep tucking in any filling trying to escape. Then to the left, to create another triangle, then down again, then across to finish at the bottom. Tuck in any loose ends and seal with oil.
10. Repeat with the other strips of filo and pop onto the lined baking tray.
11. Brush with a little more oil (and sprinkle with onion seeds if you fancy) then bake for 15–20 minutes.
12. Serve with Greek yoghurt mixed with a little mango chutney, if you like.

For babies and young children: The corners of the samosas can be a little crispy, so aren't ideal for little children. Simply cut off any sharp corners before giving them to littler ones.

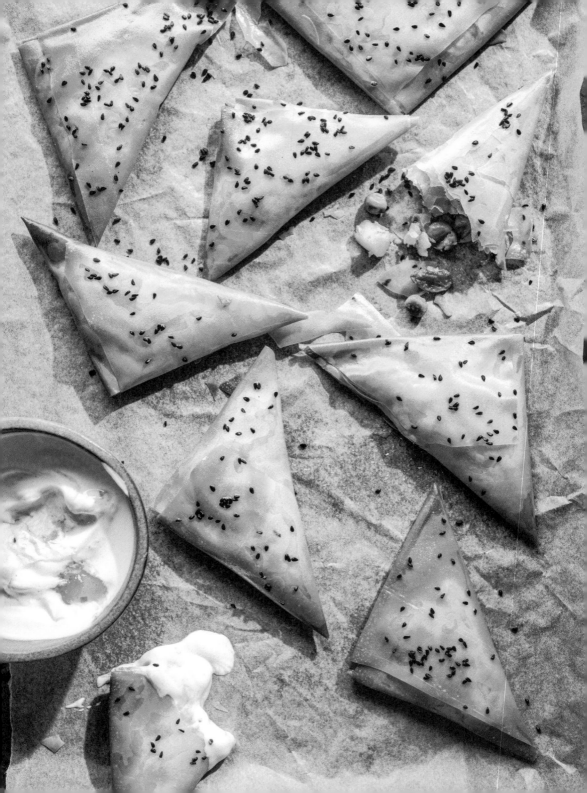

ALL-PURPOSE QUICK PASTRY

An easy shortcrust pastry recipe as an alternative to the ready-rolled stuff and without any added salt! If you're short of time you can easily use shop-bought, of course, but sometimes it's nice to make your own. This recipe is perfect for the strawberry tarts on page 197 and the jam on page 203. You can also use it to top pies (like the Green Veg and Lentil Pie, page 155).

Makes: 350g pastry
Prep time: 15 minutes, plus chilling time.

200g plain flour
80g butter, cold, cubed
3–4 tbsp ice-cold water

1. In a bowl or food processor, sift in the flour. Now add the butter cubes and either rub between your fingers to get breadcrumbs or pulse the machine. This might take around 4–5 minutes if doing by hand.
2. Add 1 tablespoon at a time of cold water, and pulse again (or mix with a metal spoon to bring it together). When it looks like it is coming together, mould the pastry into a ball then flatten slightly into a round disc shape (around 14-cm wide, to make it easier to roll out later), and cover in clingfilm. Pop in the fridge for 30 minutes to rest.
3. Once chilled, roll out. This can be used for so many recipes, including lining pastry cases and topping pies, and can also be frozen.

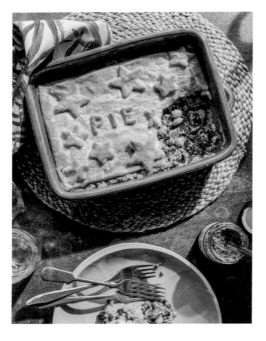

USE-UP-THE-NUTS BUTTER

In our house, nut butters are a favourite! I love this recipe – you do need a high-speed blender to ensure you get an amazing, smooth texture, but this works so well and is delicious. This is a great use of all the odds and ends of packets of nuts you have kicking about. Try to stick to the ratio of half almonds and then half the other bits and bobs and you will get a great nut butter.

Makes approx: 450g
Prep time: 10 minutes

250g almonds
250g other leftover nuts
  – peanuts, cashews, brazil, pecans
  (whatever you have in the cupboard!)
1 tbsp of veg oil

1. Preheat the oven to 200°C/180°C fan. Pop the nuts onto a large baking tray and cook for 10 mins, shaking the tray halfway through, until golden.
2. Leave to cool a little then pour into a food processor. Blend on full power for about 5 minutes. You will see it go through lots of different stages: you want the final creamy stage (so be patient!).
3. Add the oil, and blend again until combined and creamy. Scrape down the sides in the middle if need be, and make sure you have a lovely consistency.
4. Store in a sealed container or sterilised jars in the fridge for up to 2 weeks.

PEA AND MINT DIP

Makes: 350g
Prep time: 10 minutes

Pea and mint dip has been something that my mum has made for years. We have it on toast with a little garlic and a drizzle of oil. This is my version: spread it on toast, offer it with veggie sticks or dollop it on top of a salad!

 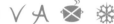

200g frozen shelled edamame
    or peas (or a mix of both!)
4 sprigs of mint, leaves picked
150g thick Greek yoghurt
1 tbsp extra virgin olive oil
juice of 1 lime or lemon
12g Parmesan (optional)

1. Put the peas or/and edamame in a colander and place under warm running water to defrost slightly, then drain and pop into a high-speed blender or food processor along with the mint, yoghurt, oil and a good squeeze of lemon juice. Blitz until combined and smooth/creamy.
2. Taste, and add a little Parmesan if you fancy.
3. Serve. It's great with carrot sticks and other crunchy vegetables, for dipping in toasted soldiers, the Samosas on page 216, or pitta.

PARMESAN, CARROT AND PARSNIP BATONS

Serves: 4–6
Prep time: 10 minutes
Cook time: 30–35 minutes

A lovely side to any meal, and these also work perfectly as starters or dipping tools. A simple way to bring a variety of super tasty veggies to the whole family.

300g carrots, peeled, quartered and
    cut into 7-cm batons
300g parsnips, quartered and cut
    into 7-cm batons
2 tbsp olive oil
15g Parmesan cheese, finely grated

1. Put a large pan of water on to boil. Preheat the oven to 200°C/180°C fan. Add the veg to the pan and simmer on the hob for 5 minutes, drain and let steam, dry for a few minutes.
2. Add to a roasting tray, drizzle with oil and roast for 20 minutes until starting to caramelise. Sprinkle over the Parmesan and toss to coat the veg, then roast for another 10–15 minutes until melted and crispy.
3. Leave to cool a little, then enjoy!

> **For babies and young children:** You might want them a little softer for young babies, so just check that they squeeze nicely between finger and thumb before offering it to them. Make sure they are nice and soft for toddlers too.

SWEET POTATO HUMMUS

Makes: 800g
Prep time: 10 minutes

We love making hummus recipes at home as they are so simple and easy to adapt. This sweet potato hummus is just a little different, with a lovely sweet taste and is great as a side to finger foods or spread on toast.

2 medium sweet potatoes (approx 450g)
400g tin of chickpeas, drained
½ a clove of garlic, peeled and
    roughly chopped
2 tbsp of tahini
juice of 1 lemon
80mls extra virgin olive oil

1. Stab the sweet potato with a fork and place in the microwave on high for 10 minutes to cook until soft and scoopable. Cut in half and leave to one side to cool a little.
2. In a food processor add the chickpeas, garlic, tahini, the lemon juice and the oil, whizz then add the cooked sweet potato (discard the skin) and whizz up again until combined.
3. Serve with veggie croutons, breadsticks, toasted pitta bread for dipping, or even spread into sandwiches as an extra flavour boost.

QUICK COCONUT FLATBREAD

Makes: 8 flatbreads
Prep time: 10 minutes
Cook time: 20 minutes

This bread is such a great addition to a main meal, use it to mop up the Cover All Curry (page 148), the dahl (page 152), or for any of the dips in this chapter!

300g self-raising flour, (wholemeal
    if possible) plus extra for dusting
150g coconut yoghurt
6 tbsps of desiccated coconut

1. In a large bowl mix the flour, coconut yoghurt and desiccated coconut with the oil and 4 tablespoons of warm water. Mix with your hands, to combine to bring it to form a dough.
2. Remove from the bowl and pop onto a flour dusted surface, kneading with your hands to bring it to more of a smooth dough.
3. Split the dough in half, then each half into 4 pieces (8 pieces in total).
4. Put a large (non-stick) pan on a high heat while you roll the dough pieces into rough 12x14cm ovals.
5. Fry in the dry pan for 1–2 minutes on each side until cooked, golden and a little charred all over.

Note: page numbers in **bold** refer to photographs.

adult nutrition 22–8
allergies 54–5
almond 203, 219
alternative ingredients 108–9
apple 72, 83
    apple crumble Bircher 112, **113**
    apple and forest fruit marzipan crumble 194
    beetroot, apple and sweet potato crisps 185
    on-the-go apple and blackberry parcel **204**, 205
    pork casserole with roast apples 174, **175**
apricot 97, 173
avocado 73, 103, 127, 156
    smashed avocado and chive toast topper 118

baby nutrition 29–32
balanced diets 13–17, 34
banana 64, 72, 111, 114
    baked banana bars 120, **121**
    banana, blueberry and nutty butter 118
    sugar-free banana custard 195
baps, monster breakfast **126**, 127
batch-cooking 27, 70, 78–9
bean(s) 17, 83, 97, 101–2, 135, 140, 160, 162, 169
    black beans 156, **157**
    cauliflower cheese and butter bean mash 214
beef, 3-way pasta sauce 166–7, **167**
beetroot
    beetroot, apple and sweet potato crisps 185
    beetroot brownie 192, **193**
Bircher, apple crumble 112, **113**
blackberry
    blackberry chia seed jam 203
    on-the-go apple and blackberry parcel **204**, 205
blueberry 73
    banana, blueberry and nutty butter 118
    blueberry breakfast muffins 114, **115**
body image 36
bread 64, 96, 103, 148, 203
breakfast 35, 102–3, 110–27
breast milk 29, 31
broccoli 72
    broccoli and fish piester bake 158, **159**
brownie, beetroot 192, **193**
budgets, cooking on 70–1
burgers, turkey 151
    roast squash tagine **172**, 173

cakes
    beetroot brownie 192, **193**
    fairy **190**, 191
    lower-sugar marble 188, **189**
    see also muffins
calcium 14, 19, 24, 25, 31

calorie intake 22
calzone pittas, stuffed 143
carbohydrates 14, 16, 18, 34, 88, 96
carrot 65, 72, 83, 138, 142, 159, 166, 178, 180, 216
    carrot, date and coconut energy balls 202
    carrot cake granola **116**, 117
    carrot and potato rostis 119
    Parmesan, carrot and parsnip batons 220
casserole, pork 174, **175**
cauliflower
    cauliflower cheese and butter bean mash 214
    Thai-style pot-roast 164, **165**
celery 72, 135, 138, 142
cheese 83, 84, 100, 103, 129, 139, 148, 168, 177–8, 210, 220
    cauliflower cheese and butter bean mash 214
    cheesy pizza muffins 208, **209**
    one-pot cheesy greens pasta 140, **141**
    simple cheesy crackers 201
    see also cream cheese; mozzarella
cheesecake bark, fruity 206, **207**
chia seed 212
    blackberry chia seed jam 203
chicken
    chicken and orzo one-pot 150
    a comforting chicken soup 138
chickpea(s) 97, 142, 159, 173, 221
children's nutrition 29–36
chocolate brownie 192, **193**
choking risk 82–3
cocoa powder 111, 188, 192
coconut (desiccated)
    carrot, date and coconut energy balls 202
    fluffy coconut pancakes 122, **123**
    quick coconut flatbread 221
coconut milk 159, 164
coconut yoghurt 130, 221
cookies, oaty 212, **213**
courgette 168, 180
    courgette fritters with minty dip 139
couscous 96, 133
crackers 96
    simple cheesy crackers 201
cream cheese 132, 162, 206
crisps, beetroot, apple and sweet potato 185
crumble
    apple crumble Bircher 112, **113**
    apple and forest fruit marzipan 194
    creamy veg **176**, 177
cucumber 72, 133, 135
curry, cover all **148**, 149
custard, sugar-free banana 195

dairy 14, 16
date, coconut and carrot energy balls 202
defrosting food 69
dhal 152, **153**
dinners 102–3, 146–83

dips 139, 220
dressings 135, 136
drinks 15, 17, 26, 33

eating, mindful 26
egg 60, 97, 100, 102–3, 127, 129, 139, 144, 151, 170, 188, 191, 208
    scrambled eggs 118
energy levels 26
equipment 106–107

fairy cakes **190**, 191
fajitas, Quorn 156, **157**
fats 17–18, 20, 31, 34
    see also oils
fibre 15, 24, 33, 39
fish 60, 84, 97, 100, 103, **134**, 135
    broccoli and fish piester bake 158, **159**
    oily 23, 24, 84
    salmon paté on toast 132
    tomato and sardine sauce 147
    tuna orzo salad **134**, 135
flatbread, quick coconut 221
flaxseed 97
    flaxseed egg 108
flours, alternative 109
folate 14, 15, 24, 26
food labels 87
food language 50
food longevity 72–3
food preparation 81–4
food refusal 9, 30, 33, 51
food shopping 63, 70–1, 80
food texture 52
food waste 62–6
foods to avoid 82–4
formula milk 29, 31
fridges 60–1, 62
frittata, quick veggie 129
fritters, courgette 139
frozen food 67–9, 70, 74–5, 97, 111, 210
    non-freezable items 67
fruit 15–17, 23, 33–4, 60, 65, 72–3, 83, 88, 97–9, 103, 111, 198
    fruity cheesecake bark 206, **207**
    see also specific fruit

gnocchi 162, **163**
grains 100
    sweet/savoury 133, **133**
granola, carrot cake **116**, 117
Greek yoghurt 139, 188, 206, 210
green bean(s) 140, 169
guacamole 156, **157**

hanger 34
healthy eating 11–39
    obstacles to 6–9
herbs 91, 92–3, 100, 102
hummus 73, 103
    sweet potato 221

icing 191
independence 26, 35
iron, dietary 15–16, 24, 31, 33, 97

jam, blackberry chia seed 203
juices 17

lasagne, cheat's veggie 178, **179**
leek 138, 147, 174
leftovers 62–3, 71, 180
lentil(s) 97, 102, 166, 178
    green veg and lentil pie **154**, 155
    sweet potato and lentil dhal 152, **153**
lunch boxes 88–90
lunches 88–90, 102–3, 128–45

macronutrients 18
mash, cauliflower cheese and butter
bean 214
mayo, zesty 151
meal planning 27, 71, 74–5
mealtimes 26–7, 36, 41–55
    making separate meals 52–3
    obstacles to 46
measurement conversions 86
meat 23, 60, 70–1, 100, 102–3
    see also specific meats
Mediterranean-style eating 43–5
micronutrients 19
milks 29, 31, 65, 97, 100, 111–12, 120, 122,
124, 144, 177, 195, 208
minerals 14–16, 19, 24–6, 31
mood 34
mozzarella 140, 143, 178, 180
muffins
    blueberry breakfast 114, **115**
    cheesy pizza 208, **209**
mushroom 127, 143, 166, 168, 183
    creamy mushroom pancakes 144–5, **145**

noodles
    pad Thai 170, **171**
    tofu and watermelon 136
nut butter 102–3, 111, 118
    use-up-the nuts butter 219
nutrients 18–21
nutritional needs 22–37
nutritional supplements 23–5, 31
nut(s) 117, 177, 202–3, 206, 215, 219

oats 96, 103, 111–12, 117, 120, 122, 177, 194
    oaty cookie 212, **213**
oils 91, 94–5
omega-3 fatty acids 15, 23–4, 31
orangey breakfast waffles 124, **125**
organisational skills 57–103
orzo
    chicken and orzo one-pot 150
    tuna orzo salad **134**, 135

pad Thai 170, **171**
pancakes
    creamy mushroom 144–5, **145**
    fluffy coconut 122, **123**
pangrattato topping 203
Parmesan, carrot and parsnip batons 220
passata 143, 152
pasta 96, 101–3

3-way pasta sauce 166–7, **167**
broccoli and fish piester bake 158, **159**
cheat's veggie lasagne 178, **179**
one-pot cheesy greens pasta 140, **141**
see also orzo
pastry
    all-purpose quick 197, 218
    filo 216
    puff 155, 205
paté 132
peach 97
    easy peachy sponge 186, **187**
peanut butter 97, 101, 136, 170, 212
pea(s) 97, 140, 147, 169, 216
    pea and mint dip 220
pepper 73, 133, 143, 166, 180
pesto 73, 97
    pesto 3 ways 215
physical activity 27
pie, green veg and lentil **154**, 155
pittas, stuffed calzone 143
pomegranate seeds 130, 133
pork casserole with roast apples 174, **175**
porridge 112
portion sizes 38–9
potato 64, 72, 142, 180, 183, 214, 216
    carrot and potato rostis 119
poultry 60, 65, 138, 147
prawn 168–9, 170
pregnancy 24, 25
processed foods 21, 106
protein 15–16, 18, 89, 97, 103
pulses 17

Quorn fajitas 156, **157**

raisin(s) 97, 212, 216
rest 27
rice 96, 103, 133
    baked risotto 168–9, **169**
rostis 119
routines 26, 34

salads 102
    tuna orzo salad **134**, 135
salmon paté on toast 132
salt 20, 30, 52, 106
samosas, veggie 216, **217**
sauces
    3-way pasta 166–7, **167**
    tomato and sardine 147
sausage, veggie bangers & mash with
mushroom gravy **182**, 183
scones, frozen veg 210, **211**
seasonal foods 71, 98–9
seeds 83, 101, 114, 117, 120, 194, 201,
203, 212
smoothies, easy family 111
snacks 34, 102–3, 200–21
sorbet, 2-ingredient 198, **199**
soup
    a comforting chicken 138
    leftover veg 142
    Mexican tomato 160, **161**
spices 91, 92–3

spinach 72, 111, 127, 144
    creamy tomato and spinach gnocchi
    162, **163**
sponge, easy peachy 186, **187**
store-cupboard staples 96–7
strawberry 73, 206
    strawberry tarts **196**, 197
sugar 20, 23, 30, 33, 52, 106
sugary drinks 17, 33
sultana(s) 117, 120, 216
sweet potato 142, 178
    beetroot, apple and sweet potato
    crisps 185
    sweet potato hummus 221
    sweet potato and lentil dhal 152, **153**
sweetcorn 143, 208

tagine, roast squash **172**, 173
tarts, strawberry **196**, 197
teenage nutrition 33–6
toast 102
    easy toast toppers 118
    salmon paté on toast 132
toddler nutrition 29–32
tofu 100
    coronation tofu wrap 130, **131**
    tofu and watermelon noodles 136
tomato 64, 83, 127, 143, 156, 168–9, 173,
178, 180, 208
    creamy tomato and spinach gnocchi
    162, **163**
    Mexican tomato soup 160, **161**
    simple tomato sauce 166–7
    tomato and sardine sauce 147
tuna orzo salad **134**, 135
turkey burger 151

varied diets 13, 17
vegan diets 25, 31
vegetables 15–17, 23, 33–4, 60–1, 65, 72–3,
83, 88, 97–9, 101–3
    acceptance 48–9
    budgets 70–1
    leftover veg traybake 180, **181**
    see also specific vegetables
vitamins 14–15, 19, 25, 26

waffles, orangey breakfast 124, **125**
water intake 15, 17, 26
watermelon and tofu noodles 136
weaning 29
wholegrains 14, 23–4, 29, 103
wraps, coronation tofu 130, **131**

yoghurt 103, 112, 139, 151, 198
    see also coconut yoghurt; Greek
    yoghurt

Saying thank you to all the people who have helped me with this book feels a little like an overwhelming task – I think I could fill an entire book with names. But I want to first thank Joe Wicks, without his generosity, support and mentoring, I wouldn't be here today with three books to my name. I'll be forever grateful. I'm also so thankful to everyone at Bev James Management, I'm honoured to be a part of your team.

I also must thank the amazing team at Ebury. Sam, Jess, Rachel and especially Anya, who kept it together through ALL of my very particular requests for this book! It is so wonderful to be a part of the Ebury family.

The work from others that has gone into this book has been incredible too. Lucy the designer, Julia my editor, Liz and Max the photographers and Frankie and Christina the food stylists. Your skills are incredible, thank you for bringing my recipes and words to life in this book. A huge thank you to Christina, who helped me get the recipes just right, I'm so grateful to you and so proud of what we've created, along with Rebecca who helped with the early recipe creations too.

I have to thank Olivia, Sara and especially Laura Matthews for recipe testing for me – thanks for your feedback, for helping to finesse these recipes to make them as delicious and healthy as possible. My family and friends have helped hugely too – Kristina (my sister), my parents, in laws and all those who have tasted the recipes for me along the way. It's been a collaboration!

Of course I have to thank my husband, Danny and my two kiddos – Adaline and Rafael for being chief taste testers. You both do so much to help me, without even knowing it. Thank you and thanks Ada for giving me a real challenge by rejecting many a meal on first go… I'm sure it helped in the long-run! I'm very lucky to be surrounded by all of these incredible people.

1

Vermilion, an imprint of Ebury Publishing,
20 Vauxhall Bridge Road,
London SW1V 2SA

Vermilion is part of the Penguin Random House group of companies whose addresses can be found at global.penguinrandomhouse.com

Penguin
Random House
UK

Copyright © Charlotte Stirling-Reed 2023
Photography © Haarala Hamilton 2023

Charlotte Stirling-Reed has asserted her right to be identified as the author of this Work in accordance with the Copyright, Designs and Patents Act 1988

First published by Vermilion in 2023

www.penguin.co.uk

A CIP catalogue record for this book is available from the British Library

Commissioning Editor: Sam Jackson
Project Editor: Anya Hayes
Editor: Julia Kellaway
Designer: Studio Polka
Photographer: Haarala Hamilton
Food & Prop Stylists: Frankie Unsworth and Christina Mackenzie

ISBN 9781785044045

Printed and bound in Italy by L.E.G.O S.p.A.

The authorised representative in the EEA is Penguin Random House Ireland, Morrison Chambers, 32 Nassau Street, Dublin D02 YH68.

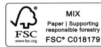

MIX
Paper | Supporting responsible forestry
FSC® C018179

Penguin Random House is committed to a sustainable future for our business, our readers and our planet. This book is made from Forest Stewardship Council® certified paper.

The information in this book has been compiled as general guidance on the specific subjects addressed. It is not a substitute and not to be relied on for medical, healthcare or pharmaceutical professional advice. Please consult your GP before changing, stopping or starting any medical treatment. So far as the author is aware the information given is correct and up to date as at March 2023. Practice, laws and regulations all change and the reader should obtain up-to-date professional advice on any such issues. The author and publishers disclaim, as far as the law allows, any liability arising directly or indirectly from the use or misuse of the information contained in this book.